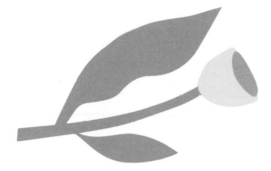

FRESH FACE

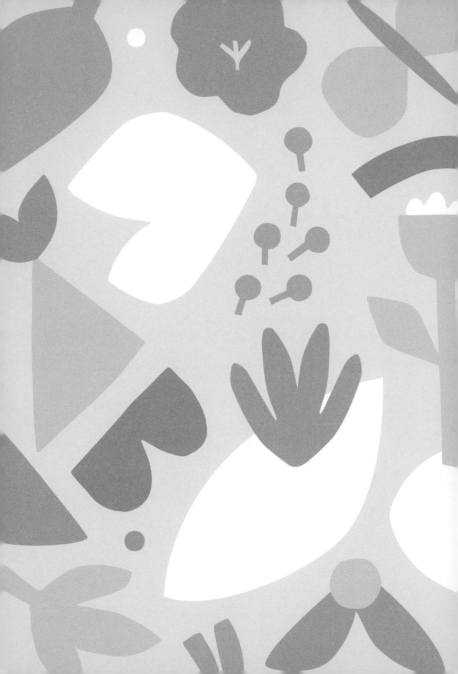

FRESH FACE

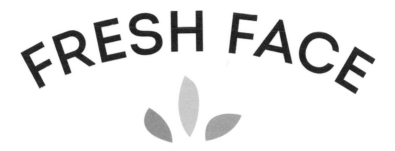

Simple routines for beautiful glowing skin, every day

MANDI NYAMBI, M.S.
illustrated by MYRIAM VAN NESTE

CHRONICLE BOOKS
SAN FRANCISCO

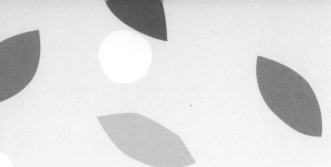

Library of Congress Cataloging-in-Publication Data:
Names: Nyambi, Mandi, author.
Title: Fresh face / Mandi Nyambi, M.S.
Description: San Francisco : Chronicle Books, [2019]
Identifiers: LCCN 2018043659 | ISBN 9781452178400 (pbk. : alk. paper)
Subjects: LCSH: Face--Care and hygiene. | Skin--Care and hygiene. | Beauty,
Personal.
Classification: LCC RL87 .N93 2019 | DDC 646.7/2--dc23 LC record available at
https://lccn.loc.gov/2018043659

Manufactured in China.

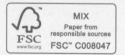

Design by Abbie Goveia.

10 9 8 7 6 5 4 3 2 1

Chronicle books and gifts are available at special quantity discounts to corporations, professional
associations, literacy programs, and other organizations. For details and discount information, please
contact our corporate/premiums department at corporatesales@chroniclebooks.com or at
1-800-759-0190.

Chronicle Books LLC
680 Second Street
San Francisco, California 94107

www.chroniclebooks.com

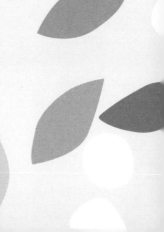

"That's the number one thing you have to do,
is to work on yourself and to fill yourself up
and keep your cup full." –Oprah

For all those looking for a fresh start and a path to glow.

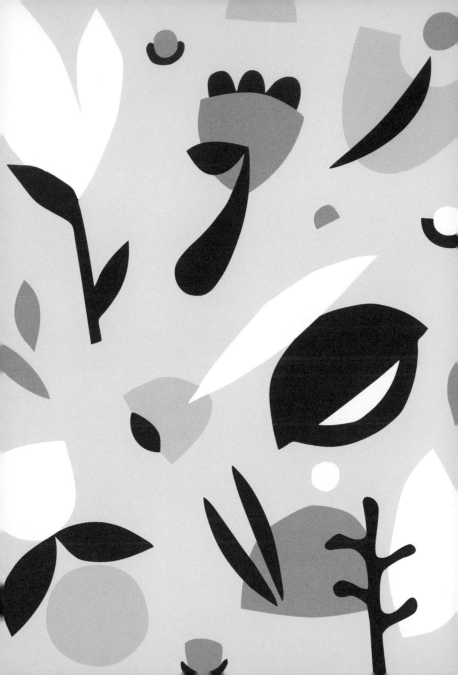

Contents

Introduction

A good skin-care routine should tend to your spirit, your mental pleasure zones, and your skin. Your body is an interconnected system, and how you feel shows up in so many parts of you. The way you treat yourself can radically change the way your soul and psyche are fed. If you're like me, skin care is not just about managing blemishes. Sometimes it's a coping mechanism, and most of the time it's a means of survival. It gets you through those midday meetings rife with mansplaining, prepares you for a big date, and heals you after an all-out weekend festival. I began to fully unlock those treasures once I developed a personal playbook.

I used to set aside time and plan for my self-care routine. While this is necessary to a degree, I found myself getting bogged down in calendar slots and feeling guilty if I wasn't able to make room for a session on a consistent basis. My first mistake: self-care shouldn't be a burden to my schedule. My second mistake: too many rules and a narrow view about what self-care needed to look like in my home.

I firmly believe that you don't have to spend a lot of money or change your entire life to have great skin. You shouldn't have to change yourself to be beautiful. That's not a cliché, that's just a fact. This book is about staying who you are and working toward the skin you've always dreamed of. You'll read about the little things you can do to get there.

Building a healthy relationship with your skin takes work and time. Not to personify it to oblivion, but your skin has needs! When you have dark circles under your eyes, you put on concealer—but what about minimizing those dark circles in the first place? How about when you break out spontaneously, or when you find flaky patches on your forehead? If you're like I used to be, you probably just groan in the mirror and try to cover it up. Well, that all changes today!

Think of this book as the ultimate every-person guide to navigating your skin-care journey. There's a routine for all the wacky and mundane scenarios in life, so you don't have to be concerned about how to work skin care into your day-to-day. Don't worry about it; just flip to the routine designed for the moment/freak-out that you're having.

I wrote this book because I think skin care can be accessible to everyone if they're given the right tools. In return, I hope you'll dedicate more time to yourself. Not just investing in the way you look, but also in how you feel about your well-being. Let me meet you where you are in your self-care journey and take you where you want to go. I'm not asking you to go out and buy expensive crystals, though you can if you want to, or telling you to book a monthly facial, although you can never go wrong with a little luxury. Instead, I'm recommending that you carry a mist spray in your purse for when you need a boost and suggesting that you create space for your skin-care routine in your home. And if you're an overachiever, you'll set a bedtime for yourself, because there's nothing like a good night of beauty sleep. You just can't put beauty sleep in a bottle, though some have tried.

THE ASSUMPTIONS THAT INFORM THIS BOOK

ALL SKIN IS NOT CREATED EQUAL.

WE ALL HAVE THE CAPACITY FOR BEAUTIFUL SKIN.

WE CAN TAKE CONTROL OF OUR SKIN GOALS.

WE KNOW OUR BODIES AND OUR SKIN BEST.

ANYONE CAN BE A SKIN-CARE GURU.

EVERYONE DESERVES THE TOOLS TO MAKE THEMSELVES FEEL HEALTHY AND BEAUTIFUL.

WE ARE CONSTANTLY MOVING TOWARD BECOMING THE BEST VERSIONS OF OURSELVES.

WE ALL DESERVE A LOVING RELATIONSHIP WITH OUR SKIN.

ATTACKING OUR SKIN IS A FORM OF ATTACKING OURSELVES.

WE LIVE OUR LIVES IN OUR SKIN, AND THAT'S WHY SELF-CARE MATTERS.

Each routine presented in this book focuses on a specific skin concern and the ingredients to seek out in order to manage it. You won't find mentions of any brands or specific product shout-outs because my only loyalty is to having beautiful, healthy skin. Everything you'll read is based on the latest research in dermatology and skin care, interviews with dermatologists, and what I've learned from my own personal explorations.

There are all kinds of routines in here to accommodate any lifestyle. Whether you have sensitive skin or a crazy travel schedule, or you're a self-care maven, there's something in here for you. The routines are all relatively simple to do, and you don't need extravagant supplies, crazy tricks, or hours every day to have glowing skin. The point is, anyone can do this. Let go of all your anxiety and open yourself up to *finally* taking care of your skin.

Expand your mind, because I'll show you how to bring your skin-care routine into public bathroom stalls, airplane seats, office cubicles, and anywhere else life takes you.

My only hope is that this book will inspire you to fit your skin into the context of your life. Just like your skin, your life changes, and the scenarios I present here morph so you can tailor them to your needs. The most important thing is that you give your skin a voice and lend it your ear. Listen to what it tells you by simply paying attention.

Love your skin, and accept it as it is in this moment. Here's to a fresh start.

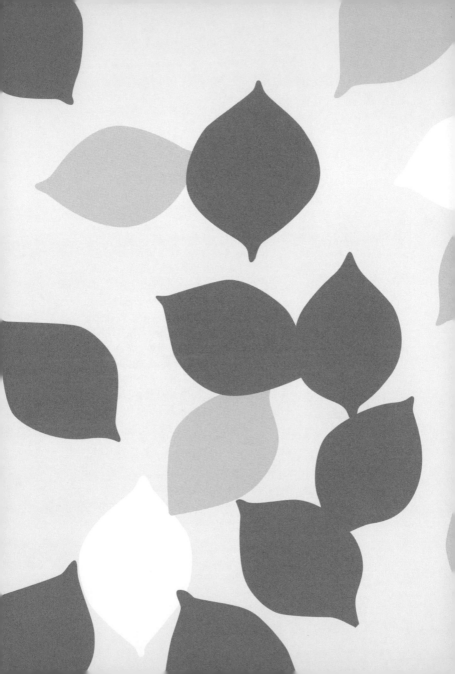

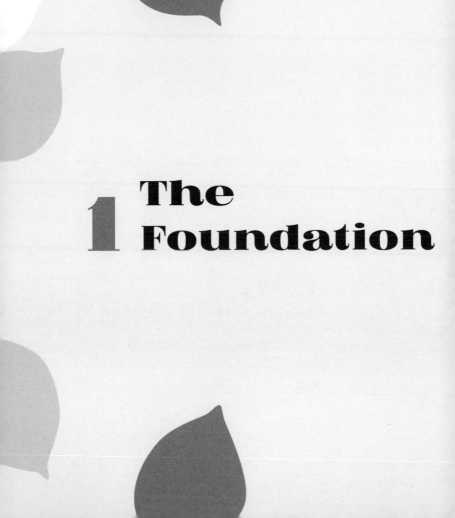

1 The Foundation

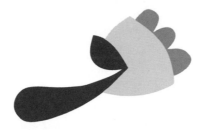

ANATOMY OF THE SKIN

We are all intimately familiar with what it means to live in skin. It's the protective barrier that allows us to plunge into any adventure without fear of harming our warm and mushy insides. It is the communication channel to our inner parts, letting us know with irritated bumps when we've eaten something bad or that we're scared or that our skin is drying out. There are so many complex layers to the skin, and understanding what those are will help you understand your skin and yourself a bit better.

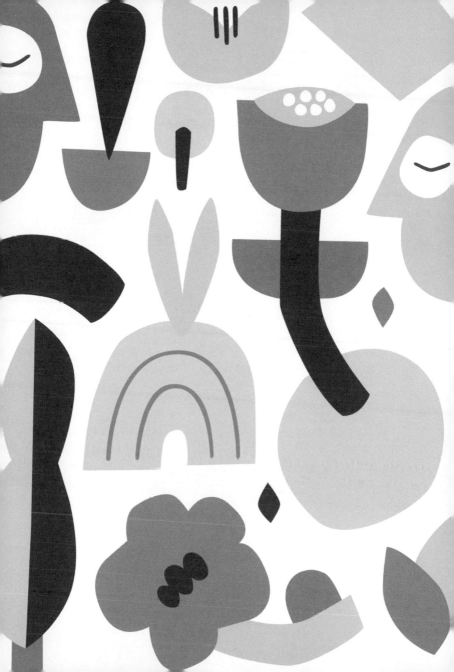

There Are Layers to This

The skin has three layers: the innermost *hypodermis,* the *dermis,* and the *epidermis,* the outermost layer. In the hypodermis, the fatty layer, you find connective tissues that provide the structure and integrity of the skin, and blood vessels that facilitate the transport of nutrients and waste from the inside of the body to the outside, and vice versa. Sweat glands are also found here and draw a salty solution to the surface of your skin through the dermis and the epidermis.

The dermis is a mixture of sweat glands, nerve endings, hair follicles, and sebaceous glands, which produce *sebum,* lubricating oils secreted by the skin's sebaceous glands.

On the very top is the epidermis, the layer we are all most familiar with. It contains the pigment-producing melanocytes and acts as a tough waterproof barrier to the outside world. It also contains the *stratum corneum,* or the skin's protective layer, which is a wall of dried-out cells and a matrix of lipids. All together, it plays a central role in water retention and preventing moisture loss. When this barrier is compromised, you experience symptoms such as sensitive skin, dry skin, and even acne lesions. It's important to use products that will help build up your skin's barrier in addition to controlling symptoms to truly heal your skin.

When trying to improve the quality of your skin with the foods you eat or the products you slather on, you have to understand how the skin's network of cells, hair, and microbes work in order to get the best results. The closer a product is to your skin, the deeper it will penetrate.

The Ecology of the Skin

The *skin microbiome* is the ecosystem of microorganisms, including bacteria, yeast, and viruses, that live in and around the surface of the skin. The bacteria that live in the human body outnumber our human cells 10 to 1, so in many ways, we are earth-dwelling cyborgs that are more bacteria than human. The skin microbiome is made up of millions of bacteria that are constantly fighting for equilibrium. These bacteria do everything from maintaining a healthy skin barrier to locking in moisture to protecting against pathogens and preventing acne. Bacteria play a big role in your skin health, so using a probiotic in your routine will maintain this incredible army of skin-supporting agents.

We each have a unique skin ecosystem, so unique, in fact, that forensic scientists can use it like a fingerprint to tell you apart from someone else. So don't leave your used face cloth at a crime scene. When you're using products that are "antibacterial" or "antimicrobial," you're not just wiping out important microbial friends, you're stripping away part of your identity. This is all to say that we have very different skin ecosystems from one another, so products may vary in efficacy, and it's important to listen to what your skin is telling you. As you go through the routines later in the book, try different combinations based on what your skin needs at any given moment.

The microbiome is perhaps the latest frontier in skin care, and new information about how important it is for us to maintain a healthy skin microbiome continues to emerge.

What we do know is that diversity is an important marker for making sure that our *skin flora,* the collection of bacteria and microorganisms that live on the skin's surface, is in good shape. No matter what skin condition you might have, the common denominator is that people with acne, rosacea, dry skin—you name it—all have a low diversity of bacteria. This is one form of *dysbiosis*, or an imbalance in the skin microbiome, which typically happens as a result of using too many antimicrobial or antibacterial products. A more diverse skin microbiome is tied to better moisture retention, less extreme eczema, fewer acne lesions, and a healthy skin barrier. One of the most important changes you can make to achieve the skin you want is to think about how your routine affects your skin's ecosystem.

The road to skin wellness looks a lot messier than we originally thought. British fashion designer Vivienne Westwood showers once a week to stay beautiful. She's convinced that keeping the natural flora on her skin is the best way to reach her skin goals. She's not alone in this thinking. In fact, the traditional ways of managing acne, like using antibiotics, are starting to lose their effect and their favor because bacteria are fighting back. When you use antibiotics, you indiscriminately eliminate whole swaths of your microbiome. The downside is that the bacteria that persist are resistant to those antibiotics, and when there's no competition left, they take over. This creates a dangerous situation: 1) our antibiotics can't stop those bacteria from doing harm, and 2) the bacteria that would have naturally kept these superbugs in check have now been eliminated.

Acne is caused by *Propionibacterium acnes*, so the field of dermatology has worked very hard to get rid of this bacteria from our skin. The problem is that we actually need *P. acnes* to help fight against other pathogenic bacteria. Acne makes up 60 percent of your skin microbiome. Some daring scientists are putting acne bacteria back on the face and seeing positive results in flare-ups and lesions on their patients. Their research shows that there are some strains of *P. acnes* that help prevent breakouts. Yeah, you read that right. This may sound sacrilegious, so take a seat. From now on, don't worry about eliminating bacteria on your face; instead you need to grow lots of it if you want clear, healthy skin.

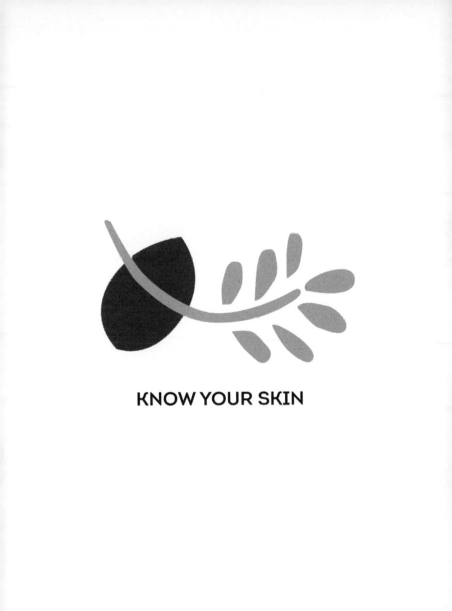

KNOW YOUR SKIN

Dealing with Skin Concerns

Before you launch into the routines and wealth of information in this book, you'll need to start with a rough assessment of your skin. How do you classify your skin? Is it rough, oily, sensitive, or pigmented? These are some of the characteristics that will help you whittle down which routines will work best for you and your needs. I've come up with a few general breakdowns and guidelines for the most common skin concerns. You may find that you're a combination of a few, or maybe you'll fall squarely in one category. Take a minute to get up close and personal with your skin and check in with what it needs from you.

Dry Skin

Dry skin has its unique challenges, including flakiness, tightness, irritation, inflammation, and redness. As you know, dry skin can cause physical discomfort, making you hyperaware of your skin's texture. So when it comes to your skin care, half the time it's about relieving those symptoms of discomfort. I get it. But let's take it a step further and talk about some ingredient guidelines to help you face seasonal challenges. During the winter months, you'll want to apply an extra layer of moisturizer or use a heavy cream to ensure that you don't lose moisture to harsh winds. You may want to moisturize more than once a day to keep up with the hydration needs of your skin.

During the transitional seasons (fall and spring), you'll need to take things day by day. I recommend checking the weather to see if your environment will be more windy or mild. When things heat up outside, you'll have to contend with air conditioners inside. While they can provide relief from the heat of the sun, they are also extremely drying to the skin. Don't skip that moisturizing step in the summer; instead you can opt for a hydrating serum in addition to a light moisturizer. You always have options.

Oily Skin

Oily skin can create a constant quest for balance. It's more than just sweating a lot when doing physical activity; it's feeling a layer of grease on your skin even in dry environments. To be clear, you absolutely need oil on your skin to keep it healthy, but just how much is hard to figure out. Thankfully, there are some signs you can look to for guidance, like acne. Excess sebum creates the perfect environment for bacteria to grow, thrive, and wreak havoc. Not all bacteria are bad, but *P. acnes*, the bacterium most closely associated with acne, does find a happy home in an oily environment. So when you're thinking about managing oily skin, you also need to think about balancing the production of oils and sebum on the face as part of your blemish care.

When managing oily skin, it helps to investigate the *comedogenicity* of a product's ingredients. A comedogenic ingredient is one that is more likely to clog your pores, but it's not a zero-sum game. The scale of comedogenic oils is a very helpful tool for picking out the right products for your skin, which may be more acne prone in addition to being oily. A rating of 0 on the comedogenic scale indicates an incredibly low probability, if any, that the skin-care product will clog pores and lead to a breakout, whereas a 5 is a breakout guarantee and can't be tolerated by even the driest of skin types.

COMEDOGENICITY	INGREDIENT
0	ARGAN OIL HEMPSEED OIL
1	SHEA BUTTER CASTOR OIL GRAPE SEED OIL ROSEHIP OIL
2	SHEA BUTTER JOJOBA OIL OLIVE OIL PUMPKIN SEED OIL
3	AVOCADO OIL SESAME OIL
4	COCOA BUTTER COCONUT OIL RED PALM OIL
5	WHEAT GERM OIL

Combination Skin

There's no cut-and-dried rule for determining if you have combination skin. Even when we very clearly have just dry or oily skin, most of us deal with more than one skin issue, sometimes at the same time. In the case of combination skin, we're talking about a situation where some areas of the face are usually dry and other areas are usually oily. One typical example is having a very oily T-zone but dry skin around the rest of the face. Product decisions tend to be a little more difficult when you're dealing with two types of skin textures, but paying close attention to the comedogenicity scale and making sure to moisturize even in the T-zone is a good place to start.

Hyperpigmentation

Everyone is susceptible to hyperpigmentation because we all produce a pigment called *melanin*. It's the same pigment that gives us our unique hues, from light to dark skin. Our skin tone is a reflection of how much melanin our skin cells produce. It is most popularly known for its photoprotective qualities—it's a biological sunscreen that works by absorbing UV rays. Melanin is also a great scavenger of free radicals that wreak havoc below the skin's surface.

We know that high melanin content and dark skin correlate with reduced signs of aging, lower rates of skin cancer, and increased photoprotection when compared to people with fair skin. But when it comes to hyperpigmentation, all of those benefits of melanin seem to wither away. In fact, hyperpigmentation is exacerbated by sun exposure, and in some instances, hyperpigmented skin is an indication of melanoma. More often than not, you'll experience hyperpigmentation from acne scars or some other minor scratches and blemishes. Regardless of your skin's complexion, you can recognize hyperpigmentation as dark and concentrated areas on the skin. A beauty mark is another form of hyperpigmentation.

There are two main methods for managing hyperpigmentation. The first is to prevent it from happening in the first place. That means taking care of your acne without popping pimples or exfoliating too often and causing damage to the skin. It also requires that you apply sunscreen daily, so that the scars left behind from a breakout don't become too concentrated by the sun's rays. Exfoliating is the next approach. Once you already have a dark spot, the pigment is several layers deep into your skin. In order to reduce the dark spot, you'll have to systematically work through those layers as the cells reach the surface and flake off. If you don't use sunscreen, the UV rays will actually induce the pigment to dive deeper into your skin. It can take up to 6 months to get rid of a dark spot, so you want to be diligent about care.

Sensitive Skin Care

There is no hard and fast definition of what sensitive skin is, which makes it even harder to manage. The most commonly accepted understanding is that sensitive skin leads to itching, irritation, burning, and stinging when the skin is exposed to external factors like skin-care products and cosmetics. Brands love to create "sensitive skin" lines to market to people who feel they have special needs. Ultimately, each of us has certain skin sensitivities, with ingredients that we tolerate and others that we just don't. The benefit of sensitive skin products is that their formulations tend to contain less abrasive ingredients. But again, this can vary widely and isn't always the case. I've seen alcohols used in sensitive skin products, and that is one of the most infamous culprits of causing irritation in people with sensitive skin.

I don't want to prescribe a list of sensitive, skin-friendly ingredients because that list won't apply to everyone and would be misleading. What I can say is that there are certain factors you can look out for, like how comedogenic an ingredient is, how complex a formulation is, and whether or not you can pronounce all of the ingredients. When it comes to avoiding extreme sensitivity, a less-is-more approach will almost certainly steer you in the right direction.

There are a few factors that contribute to the sensitivity of the skin, but ultimately it comes down to the integrity of the skin's barrier. Remember, this is the special top layer (the epidermis) that keeps your skin hydrated by preventing water loss and protecting your skin from being penetrated by harmful chemicals and physical factors. An impaired skin barrier will increase the hyperactivity of your skin and its subsequent reaction to products. You end up losing water, and when the integrity of the barrier is compromised, your skin basically has an allergic reaction to the products you put on it. If you have sensitive skin, you will want to focus on building up that barrier by exfoliating less, using gentle cleansers, applying the right nutrients, moisturizing often, and using sunscreen.

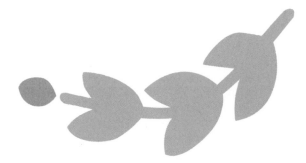

DETERMINING YOUR SKIN GOALS

When you think about what you look like on your best day—
not what you see in the mirror, but the vision you have in your
head—what do you see? What are you wearing? How is your
hair done? What does your skin look like? I've said it before:
Your skin speaks to you using its own language. It's a dynamic,
living, breathing organ that reflects who you are. So when
you think about your skin goals, you need to also think about
how they fit into your other personal goals. Do you have a lot
of stress in your life, or do you keep it more low-key? Do you
have time to commit to skin care as a hobby, or do you want
to keep it to a minimum while still reaping the benefits?

Before you set your skin goals, let's think about where your skin is today. We've talked about dry skin, oily skin, acne-prone skin, and the different signs that come along with them. In the end, we all experience a combination of those signs, though some may be more apparent than others. Think about the typical state of your skin on a daily basis and the signals it gives you throughout the day when it's not looking its best. They might be breakouts, an oily sheen, dry patches, rosacea, tightness, or any other physical signs that things are not right. Then think about how those things pop up in the course of a week, or a month, and how they change each season.

OK, so you know the signs. But how often are you aware of them as they arise? How often do you know how to respond to them? When do some of these signs start to present themselves? You can see where I'm headed with this. I'm talking about listening to your skin and finding the right way to respond to it. No matter what your dream goal is, listening to your skin will be part of making that dream the real you.

Getting a routine going will make achieving your goals a lot more realistic. It's always better to play an active role in your skin care, and not a reactive one. The next couple of sections will cover just that.

Based on your skin concerns and what your skin is telling you, think about what you want to change, improve, or just maintain in your skin. Knowing that will help direct you to the routines that will be most helpful in reaching your goals. And don't forget the routines that focus on your emotional well-being—using skin care to improve your mental health is important too.

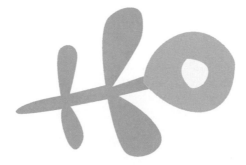

CREATING SPACE FOR YOUR SKIN

Our schedules are constantly changing, so we can't always rely on having a set time every day for our skin, but we can make sure that we have the tools and space for one.

Setting the Mood

When picking the right elements for your space, use your five senses to guide your interior design decisions. Starting with visual cues, think about what objects, colors, and aesthetics inspire you or relax you. Plants are a great way to breathe life into a space while freshening the air. Their variety of colors, sizes, and shapes create endless possibilities for decorating. Growing up, my mom and I collected seashells that we stored in colored jars in the bathroom. Each time I looked up at them, I could envision the ocean and the waves that crashed on the shores where we found them. They served as visual cues that instantly relaxed me when I stepped into my bathroom. Consider which props or elements you can bring into your self-care space that set the mood.

Chromotherapy is the branch of psychotherapy that uses the power of colors to impact our moods, emotions, and overall health. We are visual beings who internalize the cues being given by our outside environments, and color does that by sending neural messages. If painting a wall is not in your skill set, putting up a framed photograph or poster with colors that inspire and center you will be a constant visual cue you can associate with self-care. You can also use a colored lightbulb to change the whole mood of a room, from doctor's-office white to the gentle waves of Mediterranean blue.

I like to set the mood with a candle or by burning some incense. Palo santo wood burning is another popular ritual that marks a space as yours for dedicating time to yourself. And when you're done, you can close out by extinguishing the candle.

Location, Location, Location

While bathrooms are a common place for self-care, like bathing and plucking, there are other rooms in your house that can serve as special beauty sanctums. In fact, I challenge you to find one other nook in your home that can be partially dedicated to a step in your daily routine. Your favorite chaise longue can be your new masking suite. The kitchen window with the best view can be the space where you wipe your face with a moist towel before applying your evening serum. Creating physical boundaries will only limit your practice of self-care. Open up your spaces to the possibility of your wants and needs, and you'll start to see that same effect carry over into your mindset.

Keep Your Tools Clean

This may go without saying, but your tools are essential for achieving your skin goals. Fresh face towels to wipe your face in between steps of a routine are a must. You'll want to make sure you are washing your towels at least once a week. They tend to collect the grime and dirt from our faces, so wiping your face with a dirty towel erases all the hard work you put in beforehand. If you're using mask brushes, exfoliating gloves, sponges, or other tools to apply products or cleanse your skin, give those a cleaning at least once a week too.

Set Aside Time

You live in your skin every day, so it deserves some of your attention every day. Create a plan for how you're going to take care of your skin's needs in the mornings and evenings, weekends and weekdays. Think about when you can carve out time to clean your skin and when you can find a moment to mask, then sketch out a quick weekly plan. You may already do this in the context of meal prepping to eat healthier. Give your skin the same consideration.

Here are a few ways to take time for self-care no matter how busy your schedule.

DEEP CLEANSING BEFORE BED: After a long day of fighting the elements, and maybe even wearing makeup, the most important thing you can do is wash your face. Make it a luxurious moment for yourself instead of a chore.

MASK WHILE YOU GET DRESSED: Use a clay mask to reduce morning puffiness as you get dressed or while you scarf down your morning omelet.

SHEET MASK ON SUNDAYS: Set aside a specific day for sheet masking when you know you have more unstructured time. Make it a ritual and you'll start to look forward to it.

EXFOLIATE MIDWEEK: You should only exfoliate 1 to 2 times a week to remove dead cells and rejuvenate your skin. I like to do this on Wednesdays to mark the first half of the week gone and the weekend on its way.

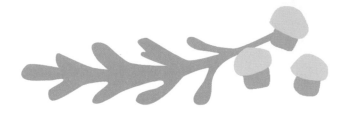

EATING FOR YOUR SKIN: THE GUT-BRAIN-SKIN CONNECTION

If your eyes are the window to your soul, then your skin is the window to your stomach—or your diet, rather. What you eat always shows up on your skin, whether in the form of an allergic reaction, pimples, or just clear skin. It all makes its way to the surface. So when searching for a more holistic way of taking care of your skin, you'll need to look beyond what you lather on your face and more closely at what you put in your mouth.

The old adage "beauty is on the inside" could not be more real, given what we now know about the importance of gut health and its impact on the skin. But it doesn't end there. Recent studies show that the gut microbiome can affect your mood as well as your skin. This two-way street also means that focusing on improving your mental health can improve your gut and skin. And when you're having skin issues, there is likely a tether to your gut that needs to be worked out. People who suffer from psoriasis also have gut issues and often find some relief in changing their diet. In this section, I'll be diving into the realm of inner beauty with a discussion about how to eat for better skin.

Sugar

Eating healthy doesn't just make you feel good; it also shows up on your skin. Having a balanced diet is one of the best ways to impact your skin. A high glycemic diet that includes processed foods, sugars, and simple carbohydrates has been found to lead to more acne on the skin. Carbohydrates from processed foods are the biggest culprits. Oprah won't give up bread for anything, and neither should you, but there are ways to have your carbs and maintain your glow. Focus on eating complex carbohydrates that are less processed and include whole grains. Avoid added sugars as best you can.

According to the United States Department of Agriculture (USDA), Americans eat about 150 pounds (60 kg) of sugar a year. For some people, that's the equivalent of their body weight. We've been conditioned to crave sugar both because of how our food is designed and because of our biology. Eating carbs in the morning will make you crave carbs all day long. So for your breakfast, steer away from refined sugars and simple carbs. Have a great green shake or a mash of banana and almond butter instead of that bagel.

Healthy Fats

Forget what your mother or your grandmother told you about avoiding fats. They were wrong. We need fats. They're not the devil, as we were taught when growing up. In fact, excess sugars are turned into fats in the body, so sugars are much more dangerous to us in some cases. The important thing is to get healthy fats into your diet, like omega-3s and omega-6s. Those are very common in nuts, superfoods like quinoa and chia seeds, and seafoods like salmon.

Water

You don't need me to tell you that drinking water is important for good skin health. You knew that before you bought this book. Here's something that you probably haven't read everywhere: TEWL. Here's the lowdown: TEWL stands for transepidermal water loss. This is the process by which water crosses the skin barrier from the inside to the outside. The speed at which this happens is a reflection of how hydrated your skin is and how well it retains moisture. You want to keep this to a minimum. Sure, water may not be that glamorous, but it is important for the vitality of your skin. You want to keep up with that water loss by drinking enough throughout the day. And if you're not going to gulp it, eat it. There are plenty of vegetables and salad leaves that have a high water content. Go for iceberg lettuce, green peppers, or cucumbers if you want to eat your water. Cantaloupe, strawberries, grapefruit, and watermelon are all fruits that have a high water content. Adding a parfait to your day will help you hydrate in a really delicious way.

The rising popularity of the gluten-free diet has less to do with celiac disease and more to do with the perceived benefits of a gluten-free diet.

It's obvious that if you have a gluten sensitivity or want to follow a gluten-free diet, you should avoid foods that contain gluten. But what about your skin-care and cosmetic products? There are a few things to consider. The gluten protein is generally too large to pass through the skin's barrier, so it is uncommon but possible for gluten in a topical application to make its way through to your bloodstream. However, about 15 to 25 percent of people with celiac disease will have a reaction to gluten in their skin-care products. In any case, a good rule of thumb is to keep any potentially gluten-containing products away from your mouth. If you don't have celiac but want to follow a strict no-gluten lifestyle, you should think about whether that will carry over into your skin-care routine. And if it does, be sure to check labels and do your research to find products that work for you.

Caveat: If you're going gluten-free, you still need to keep an eye on your overall diet. Wheat, barley, and oats are excellent sources of fiber and complete carbs, which are incredibly important for your gut health (although, unfortunately, they all contain gluten). Alternative carbs tend to be simple carbohydrates that are also high in sugar, and that kind of diet is more closely tied to outbreaks of acne. So if your goal is to have clearer skin, watch what carbs you fill up on, and find alternatives that have a high fiber content. And be mindful of your folate intake—folate is a necessary nutrient for women's health, and, at least in the United States, folate supplementation in whole grains is a significant source of dietary folate. If you're concerned about sugar, an easy way to reduce your blood sugar after a meal is to eat your proteins first, then your veggies, and then your carbs. It's as effective as many blood sugar lowering drugs.

Eat Right for Your Skin

Vitamins, nutrients, and probiotics are important for a healthy lifestyle and for maintaining healthy skin. Our bodies are very good at regulating our homeostasis, but there are elements we just can't make ourselves. In these cases, we need to supplement our diets with the vitamins that will give us that healthy glow. You can seek out these nutrients in your food or purchase them at the drugstore.

Eating for your skin should be inspired by the foods you love. There's no need to seek out obscure foods just because they have health benefits. Food is medicine, but if you don't enjoy it, it can be more like cough syrup than a healing aid. When you're eating mindfully, the experience and goal are all about achieving harmony throughout your body's ecosystem, and that translates onto the skin. Ayurvedic medicine found foods called *adaptogens* that work to achieve that harmony. Part of the power of adaptogenic foods is that they can also mitigate future stress. They are not only healing for the body but also the soul. Beauty starts from within, so here's a quick guide to some vitamins, nutrients, and adaptogens you can add to your diet that will literally leave you lit from within.

NUTRIENT	SKIN BENEFIT	FOOD SOURCE
VITAMIN A	LONGEVITY, SKIN REPAIR	FISH, EGGS, CARROTS, SPINACH, SWEET POTATOES, BEEF, DAIRY
VITAMIN B12	SKIN ELASTICITY	MEATS, POULTRY, EGGS, SHELLFISH, DAIRY
VITAMIN C	COLLAGEN FORMATION, ANTIOXIDANT	FRUITS (STRAWBERRIES, ORANGES, BLUEBERRIES) AND VEGETABLES (SPINACH, BELL PEPPERS, TOMATOES, BRUSSELS SPROUTS)
VITAMIN D	FIGHTS INFECTIONS, DEFICIENCY MAY RESULT IN ACNE	SUNSHINE, FORTIFIED FOODS (MILK, ORANGE JUICE, CEREALS)
VITAMIN E	LONGEVITY, SCAR PREVENTION, ANTIOXIDANTS KEEPS VITAMIN A LEVELS UP	ALMONDS, SUNFLOWER SEEDS, SALMON, AVOCADO, TROUT, VEGETABLE OILS
VITAMIN K	WOUND HEALING, REDUCES SCARRING, DARK CIRCLES, SPIDER VEINS	KALE, LIVER, DAIRY, BLUEBERRIES
ZINC	HEALING WOUNDS	MEAT, SHELLFISH, DAIRY, WHEAT GERM
OMEGA-3, -6, -9	MOISTURE RETENTION, SKIN BARRIER REPAIR, ELASTICITY	FLAX SEEDS, FATTY FISH, AVOCA-DOS, VEGETABLE OILS, PUMPKIN SEEDS, PISTACHIOS, WALNUTS, CHIA SEEDS, COCONUT OIL
LACTOBACILLUS	REPAIRING SKIN BARRIER GENERAL ANTI-INFLAMMATION	FERMENTED FOODS INCLUDING YOGURT AND KIMCHI
TURMERIC	REDUCES CORTICOSTERONE, BALANCES BODY ENERGY, BOOSTS IMMUNE RESPONSE	
ASHWAGANDHA	REDUCES CORTISOL LEVELS AND OIL PRODUCTION	

Getting More from Your Diet

It's not hard to get these necessary vitamins, minerals, and other nutrients into your diet. Here are a few ways to sneak them into what you're already eating.

BREAKFAST

• Add a side of kimchi or raw sauerkraut to your morning scrambled eggs for a probiotic hit.

• Chia seeds are a superfood and contain tons of protein and omega fats. Sprinkle them onto your yogurt or into your breakfast cereal. They don't have any taste, but they pack a mean crunch!

• Top your oatmeal or yogurt with blueberries and almond butter for a triple dose of vitamins C, K, and E.

LUNCH

• If you're at the salad bar and not sure what to pick, get the most out of a build-your-own bowl by going for the B.A.K.E.D. A.P.P. (bell peppers, avocado, kale, egg, dairy, almonds, pumpkin seeds, protein).

• A midday shake with ashwagandha powder will help regulate your cortisol levels if you're feeling stressed and create better hormonal balance. Step outside to enjoy this tempering potion and recollect yourself.

• Add a few tablespoons of kimchi to any rice dish to give it a sour kick and your gut a great dose of probiotics.

DINNER

- Season your salmon with turmeric, and let it marinate for 20 minutes before baking to create a super meal out of these nutrients. Turmeric will bring antioxidants to the table and pairs well with the healthy, succulent fats of the salmon.

- After dinner, brew a calming tea with red ginseng to help regulate your body's energy levels, and prepare to wind down for the evening.

- Use coconut oil when cooking your dinner instead of your typical grease to add more healthy fats to the mix; then use it as a makeup remover before bed.

SNACK

- Frozen fruit, particularly blueberries, makes the most refreshing snacks, and they're easy to carry.

- Mix coconut oil, matcha, and ashwagandha, and ditch your third cup of joe for a real kick and a skin boost.

- There's nothing like the smell of freshly popped popcorn; top it with an adaptogen like turmeric.

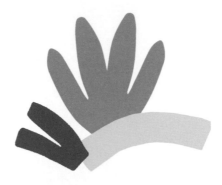

BEAUTY SLEEP

Let's talk about the fine art of sleeping with something on your face. Beauty sleep is a topic that is always hard to contend with because most of us have regally settled into our sleep routines. If you're like me, that means you basically have no sleep regimen and just pass out every night, but occasionally have your life together enough to have a routine.

A bedtime routine is in some ways more important than any other skin-care routine. At night, you have the artifacts of the day to contend with, whether that's a stain from your lunch or the smog that's settled over your pores as you maneuvered the big city. So if you prioritize anything, make it your beauty sleep.

Put Yourself to Bed

Really go the whole nine yards and tuck yourself in, read yourself a story, or listen to an audiobook.

PILLOW TALK

A silk pillow is your best bet. It doesn't crease as easily as a cotton pillow case, an important factor if you're trying to prevent fine lines from accumulating as you sleep. If you're getting 6 to 8 hours of sleep a night, you're racking up 2,500 hours of wrinkle-inducing sleep a year. Silky sheets also help prevent moisture loss, as the material is less absorbent than cotton materials. We all get dehydrated when we sleep because of how much our bodies heat up, so it's important to create an inner sanctum that helps rebalance that hydration.

HUMIDIFIER

If your inner sanctum has dry air from either a heater in the wintertime or an air conditioner in the summer, chances are your skin is parched for most of the night. A humidifier is a good investment for people who have dry skin or those who use either of these air-manipulating devices. A refreshing glass of water before bed helps as well, but the uninterrupted blast of dry air on your face as you sleep will have a really strong impact on its softness and moisture retention, and how it ages in the long run.

POSITIONS

We all have that sweet spot that plunges us right into the beautiful abyss of slumber and dreamland. If that position is not on your back, then you may want to consider a few adjustments. Sleeping on your belly causes your face to be pressed into your pillow, bearing on the weight and pressure of your head. If you're sleeping with a cotton pillow or any surface that has a lot of creases, you're imprinting that into your face, and over time those creases turn into fine lines. If you're having trouble sleeping on your back, something I struggle with personally, consider adding a few supplementary pillows to your cocoon. A back pillow to support your lower back and arch or a body pillow to prop you onto your side can help reshape your sleep position.

Masking in Your Sleep

Sleep masking is a delicate art, and I don't think that's said enough. Being coordinated and aware enough to have a mask on your face all night without getting so preoccupied that you can't fall asleep is a tricky balance. All the elements of a good night's sleep that I mentioned previously will help you optimize your sleep mask experience. Sleeping on your back allows you to keep the mask on your face and not all over your sheets. Increasing the humidity of the room will help your skin better absorb the nutrients in your mask. Choosing the right sleep mask is also important. You'll want to stay away from ingredients that might be too invigorating, so no coffee- or chocolate-infused face masks. Think of some of your favorite calming tea ingredients, like chamomile, vanilla, or even mint. These will not only bring a calming aroma to the experience but will also make you feel refreshed when you wake up in the morning.

Don't feel pressured to mask every night. One of my favorite Oscar Wilde quotes is: "All things in moderation, including moderation." So when it comes to sleep masking or any masking, take what you need, whenever you need it, and not a drop more. This is also a good time to work on any restorative initiatives you have for your face. That might include a brightening under-eye mask for reducing the appearance of dark circles. You might also consider a positive aging mask that has retinoids or collagen on the ingredients list. Your body is already doing a lot of repair work as you sleep, and collagen production is something your body focuses on during these hours. Lastly, a probiotic is a really good idea for a sleep mask, as your face is more or less undisturbed during slumber, which makes it the perfect time to work on rebalancing your skin's ecosystem after a long day.

MASK AND RELAX

Masking is the ultimate at-home skin-care ritual. There is nothing like lounging in your robe, flipping through a magazine, while soothing incense burns and your skin rejoices in a decadent mask. We have one of the biggest innovators in beauty—South Korea—to thank for bringing this practice stateside.

Ideally, we would all have started to take care of our skin from a very young age, cleansing every day and masking when needed. And while we all have a little catching up to do, masking is a great way to make up for some of the lost time. After a fresh face wash, your skin is clean and open to taking in the nutrients that a mask might contain. This is your opportunity to focus on a targeted skin-care goal, like hydration or blemish care. While there are literally hundreds of different types of face masks out there, I've highlighted a few in the following pages to help you navigate through your options. Before we dive in, here are some quick definitions to help you out.

Good for Most Skin Types

SHEET MASK

A cotton fiber sheet that is infused with a liquid or emulsion. Do not wash or rinse after use; instead, finish with a serum or moisturizer.

CLAY MASK

Typically a soothing clay-based cream that is used to dry out the skin and manage inflammation. Depending on the formulation, it can be too drying for those with already dry skin. Wash off this mask and always follow up with a moisturizer.

EXFOLIATING MASK

A chemical and/or physical exfoliant, depending on the formulation. This category of masks will help you achieve your resurfacing and longevity skin goals. Always wash off completely. Follow up with a serum for optimal absorption.

Good for Normal/Dry Skin Types

CREAM MASK

This evergreen mask typically employs moisturizing agents like oils to nourish the skin. Its light yet concentrated moisturizing abilities make this a great all-weather mask.

Good for Dry/Sensitive Skin Types

GEL MASK

This soothing and cooling mask is ideal for people with sensitive skin. It's extremely hydrating for those with dry skin, and it is collagen-boosting in certain formulations. Its light yet concentrated moisture abilities make this a mask perfect for any season.

Masking for a Cause

Brightening skin-care products are more important now in the age of extreme pollution than ever before. Soot, debris, and smog are all clinging to your pores, looking for a way in and dulling your complexion, and that is a reason to think more closely about your skin-care routine. Pollution impacts the quality of your skin and changes its complexion.

Improving your complexion with brightening products is about protecting your skin from that damage, but it should not be about changing your skin's shade. I'm disappointed by skin-care products that use brightening as a euphemism for whitening. It places artificial value on the tone or shade of one's skin, when ultimately there should be no ideal skin tone. The goal is to maintain your true complexion despite your environment.

For antipollution masks with a brightening effect, seek out those that contain vitamin C, vitamin E, and licorice root extract.

Ingredients to Know About

SNAIL MUCUS MASK

First off, ew. Yeah, I know, this is one of those ingredients you probably never thought you would be putting on your face. Just hear me out. The top three claims about snail slime are that it is moisturizing, an antioxidant, and collagen-stimulating. The goo from snails is a lubricant that helps the mollusk to safely and swiftly move from point A to point B. When applied to the face, this lubricant is a *humectant*, which means that it is able to draw water and moisture to the surface of the skin. Free radicals wreak havoc on skin when exposed to the sun and can cause damage that leads to wrinkles and fine lines. Snail slime is a pretty good antioxidant, though it's not the best. Last, but not least, some studies have shown that snail mucus can boost the production of collagen and thus the appearance of longevity.

> WHEN TO USE: The tightening effect that snail slime can have on the skin as it dries makes it a good candidate for your skin-firming needs. A snail mucus mask can be applied in the morning or in the evening, but I recommend you purchase this in a leave-in formulation, like a sheet mask.

> CAVEAT: If you're committed to a cruelty-free regimen, this ingredient is probably not for you. Mollusks could be potentially harmed in the making of these masks.

LICORICE ROOT MASK

Licorice root, scientifically known as *Glycyrrhiza glabra*, is more than just a candy flavor with a minty aftertaste. It has antipollution benefits that include neutralizing free radicals. If you're someone who spends a lot of time in the sun or lives in a very sunny climate, use a licorice root mask to mitigate the extra exposure to free radicals.

> WHEN TO USE: This is a great go-to mask after a lot of sun exposure and during the warmer months of the year. It is also a great after-blemish care mask to improve the appearance of dark spots.

VITAMIN E MASK

Vitamin E has the best antioxidant power of any vitamin, making it a great longevity ingredient, and it has a strong reputation for being moisturizing and conditioning for the skin. It comes in eight different chemical forms, the most important for the body being the tocopherol form. It is the vitamin best recognized and absorbed by our bodies. Dry skin will love the texture of vitamin E, and some studies even show that it helps temporarily improve circulation to the surface of the skin, which is also good for your hair. Consider this ingredient if hair masking is part of your self-care practice.

> WHEN TO USE: Given its very thick nature, it is best to apply a vitamin E mask at night before bed or as a sleep mask. Since your body is doing a lot of repair work, this is the right time to add vitamin E to aid in that process. If you're dealing with any scars or uneven tone, this is a great mask for managing those concerns as well.

HYALURONIC ACID MASK

A hyaluronic acid (HA) mask should be a staple in any beauty cabinet. This chemical, which is naturally found in fluids in the eye and around the knee, heart, lungs, skeletal muscles, and umbilical cord, is more than just a good moisturizing ingredient. It can also be used to heal wounds, stymie the sting of burns, and supposedly improve the appearance of wrinkles. It is perhaps most well known for being the chief molecule associated with moisture retention in the skin and throughout the body's connective tissue. Over 50 percent of the body's total HA content can be found in the skin. By binding to water molecules in the *extracellular matrix* (the space in between cells), it contributes to the integrity of the skin as well as to its hydration.

WHEN TO USE: This is an evergreen mask that is perfect for whenever your skin is feeling dry and flaky. It is also a great longevity treatment for those who want another resource for managing skin aging. I recommend using this mask in the evening before bed, though it couldn't hurt to use it as a wake-up regimen.

PROBIOTICS MASK

There are a lot of products and face regimens that aren't microbiome friendly. From using an essential oil–based serum to scrubbing our faces multiple times a day, the skin's ecosystem is constantly impacted and changed by the things we do. So it becomes essential that we also take the time to reset and rebalance that ecosystem. The skin's natural flora plays a big role in maintaining the moisture barrier, and preventing acne and rosacea flare-ups. Masking with a probiotic mask is like rolling around in the dirt, in all the best ways. Focus on masks that are water based and contain a mix of prebiotics and probiotics. *Lactobacillus* and *Bifidobacterium* are the two most common probiotics used in skin-care formulations.

> WHEN TO USE: It's always a good idea to work toward restoring the natural balance of your skin. A probiotic mask is a great treat whenever you're in skin maintenance mode. Strongly consider a mask in this category if you're experiencing symptoms like sensitive skin or a dry spell that may be the result of a disrupted skin barrier.

RUBBER MASK

I have to confess, I met the thought of letting rubber seep into my pores with great skepticism and even alarm. The benefits of doing a rubber mask are still slightly elusive to me but are worth discussing because of their growing popularity and their crossover from South Korean beauty to international infamy.

The first myth I want to clear up is that, though they may feel like it, rubber masks aren't made of rubber materials. The exact formula for each mask will vary depending on the brand and the use (e.g., hydration, blemish care), but the bases are typically made of the same material. A very common formulation is to use *alginate* (alginic acid), which is a kelp extract, as the base for the mixture. This extract is particularly deft at providing water and moisture to the skin, so rubber masks with these ingredients tend be very hydrating, soothing, and softening for the skin. The benefit difference between this type of mask and a sheet mask is that you don't lose nutrients to evaporation as the mask dries out. The entire premise is that as the "rubber" material dries and molds onto your face, the nutrients are coaxed into your pores instead of into the air.

> WHEN TO USE: Rubber masks are great for when your skin is looking dull and feeling dry, itchy, and irritated. The soothing algae base of a rubber mask will not only calm your skin but also add moisture and rejuvenate its dull appearance. Molding masks are also helpful when you feel that your skin is looking tired or puffy.

CHARCOAL MASK

Charcoal is one of those ingredients that scared us when we were young, because it meant no presents under the tree. But as you get older, you realize that 1) as an adult, you can put whatever you want under that pine, and 2) there's a lot more to this story. Charcoal was traditionally used by physicians to remove toxins from the body in the event of extreme poisoning. It is a swift and efficient way to rid the body of a systemic problem.

When it comes to skin, charcoal masks provide additional backup for removing impurities off the surface of your face and body. They are typically included in clay mask formulations as the main active ingredient.

Moderately wet an exfoliating sponge, and use it to gently rinse off your charcoal mask when you're done. This provides additional exfoliation, while taking advantage of the exfoliating qualities of charcoal.

> WHEN TO USE: Charcoal masks are useful when fighting an acne breakout or tempering oily skin. You'll want to involve this in your routine during warmer months when you are more prone to excess sweat and sebum production. When you experience a breakout, a charcoal clay mask will be very effective for drying out problem spots and reducing inflammation. When using a charcoal mask, be careful not to leave it on your face for too long. Too much drying out will actually cause mild irritation and encourage your skin to produce more sebum to make up for the lost moisture.

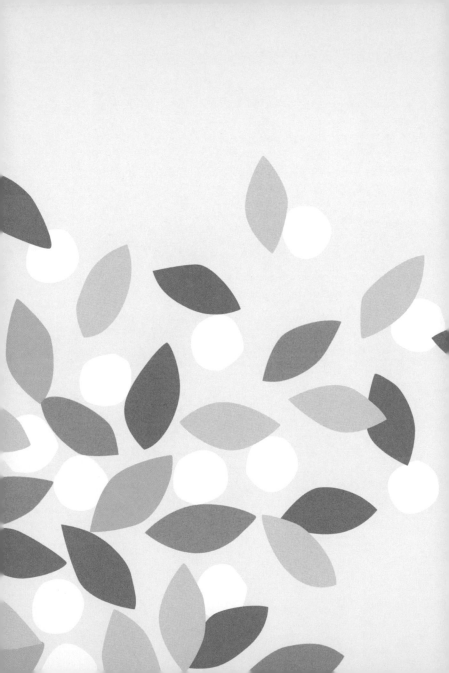

2 The Routines

Here is where the real work begins. It's Wednesday night, and you're just clearing the midweek hump. You look in the mirror, and you've got a brand-new friend on your cheek staring back at you, bathing in a dewy pool of your sebum. Not again. Not this week. We've all been there, just trying to make it to the weekend while holding it together. But what do you do next? That's where a game plan or a routine comes into play.

This section of the book is all about giving you actual tools that you can use and implement in your daily skin-care exploration. I've thought a lot about the factors in our lives that make it harder to keep a consistent skin-care routine. Wellness is all about reaching your ideal self, but I want to focus on the real and present version of you. The you that has a dog that needs to be walked before you can have your coffee in the morning, or the you that has to go to your in-laws over the holidays. Some of the routines will help you just get through the day, with on-the-go tips and tricks to find balance on your skin and in your crazy life.

I've found that starting from where you are and the life you currently lead is the best way to move toward the skin you ultimately want. How do you make gluten-free skin care work for you on a business trip? There's a routine for that. If you're coming to terms with your adult acne and just need a way to get through a week of workouts without multiple major breakouts, I have some advice on that too.

The most important thing is to stay flexible and continue to listen to your skin, as we discussed earlier. Then flip to the right page and dig in.

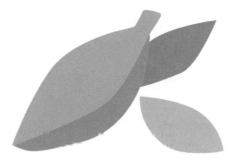

THE ANATOMY OF A ROUTINE

Before we dive into the routines that follow, here is some guidance on what a routine might contain. The steps described are ones you can build into a daily routine, beyond those described in the book. There are also some specialized steps—like applying retinol or doing a peel—that are for specific skin-care needs rather than something you should be doing every day. These steps are presented in roughly the order they should be done, so that your skin can get the most out of each ingredient. But sometimes, as you'll see in the routines that follow, it makes sense to switch things up so that you can do what's right for your skin.

Cleansing

Cleansing allows you to get past all the grime and muck of the day, the makeup and the sunscreen, right to the bare skin. That's where the magic happens. Don't think of cleansing as stripping, but more like pushing your way to the front of a crowd when you want to see what's happening up close. The type of cleanser you use should reflect your skin type and your skin needs.

OIL CLEANSER: This is a good place to start. Your face is covered in oils like sebum and other fat-soluble particles. Think back to high school chemistry: like dissolves like. Oil cleansers help to dislodge the oils and the imbedded materials within them like debris and grime.

WATER-BASED CLEANSER: Whether this is the first step of your routine or it follows an oil cleanser, the water-based cleanser is the best opportunity to remove the majority of grime from your face. A gentle water-based cleanser will go a long way to preparing your skin for the treatments to follow. This step is essential to not only giving you a clean slate to work with, but for allowing room on your face for your skin to absorb the ingredients in the rest of your products.

Water-based cleansers all work to dislodge and break up excess oils on the skin's surface. If like dissolves like, this does the opposite: it separates oil droplets from one another. If you have dry skin, then you will want to avoid an especially astringent cleanser; anything with an alcohol as an ingredient will excessively dry your skin. The goal is to dislodge excess oils without stripping them completely. That oil barrier is a mechanism of defense and is important for maintaining healthy skin.

GEL/FOAM CLEANSER: Lathering is fun. There's no doubt about that, and these cleansers are a great example of a water-based cleanser. Formulations will vary by brand, but each of them will create a nice foamy film on the surface of your skin. A good rule of thumb is to cleanse for a minute, and with a foam cleanser it's a lot easier to see exactly where you've put in elbow grease and which areas of the face need more attention. With any other cleanser that minute can seem to drag on, but this throwback to bath time should keep you occupied for a while.

POWDER CLEANSER: Those "just add water" advertisements take on new meaning with this kind of cleanser. To activate, simply add a few drops of water to a handful of powder and then work it into a lather.

BALM CLEANSER: Some classify this type of cleanser as a physical cleanser. Its thicker texture requires a bit more rubbing and working in than your typical liquid cleanser. A benefit of this is that the main cleaning action dislodges oil and dirt on the surface of your skin and may be a good option if you have combination skin.

Exfoliating

The goal of exfoliating is simple: peel back the dead layers of skin cells to give the skin a renewed glow. Exfoliation is important when you're trying to prevent and get rid of a blemish on the skin. The skin is a living organ; it's so dynamic and always changing in more ways than one. It grows by shedding, and while that may make your skin crawl, it's true. As new layers of the skin are formed, older, more external layers fall off. There are two major categories of exfoliating products: physical exfoliators and chemical exfoliators.

PHYSICAL EXFOLIATORS are just what they sound like. They're typically small grains or beads added to a solution that when rubbed into the skin will physically dislodge dead cells and resurface your face. They are a safe at-home exfoliating treatment and can be used on any kind of skin.

CHEMICAL EXFOLIATORS like peels are solutions with astringent chemicals like alpha hydroxy acids (AHAs) and beta hydroxy acids (BHAs). They basically disrupt the binding agents that connect your dead cells to the living parts of your skin. Not only do they resurface your skin, but they also brighten your complexion.

Toning

Toners are a bit of a black box in the context of a skin-care routine. They're not quite a serum and they're not quite a mask, and some of them wash off despite not being a cleanser. In many ways they're that extra *je ne sais quoi* to get the job done. Toners are typically water-based solutions with targeted active ingredients for improving the skin.

Applying Serums

Usually this step in the routine is overlooked. But serums can be an incredibly powerful source of nutrients and minerals for our skin. They are typically concentrated oils with one major ingredient, ranging from moisturizing agents to vitamin-boosting agents. You'll want to use these after you cleanse and exfoliate, to ensure that you apply them as close to the surface of the skin as possible.

Masking

Face masks are semi-intensive full-face treatments that have played a part in skin-care culture around the world for centuries. In India turmeric mask recipes are as guarded as your midwestern family casserole recipe. Think of them as a deep conditioner for your face, a period when you can deliver specific nutrients that your skin needs. There are so many different ways to mask, whether it's a sheet mask or a rubber mask or a sleep mask. I can't say enough about masks, so I wrote a whole section about them starting on page 49.

Moisturizing

Growing up, my mom checked two things before I left the house for school in the morning: 1) Did I have my homework? and 2) Did I remember to moisturize my face? Number 2 is absolutely essential no matter what kind of skin you have. Just as your body needs water, your skin needs to be hydrated from the inside and the outside. There is an endless supply of moisturizing options on the market, and you have to try a few to figure out what works best for you. There are gel moisturizers and cream moisturizers, and either one is great for oily or combination skin. Balms and butters are much thicker and may be best suited for dry skin. You should moisturize at least twice a day, once before you leave the house, and again before going to bed. During the day you battle the elements, and at night your body heats up and gets dehydrated, so there is really no skipping this step.

Applying Sunscreen

While it wasn't always cool to be the kid with white streaks of sunblock smeared all over your body, it's the number one skincare product that will keep you looking young. The Big C is scary, and you don't need me to tell you that sun damage can lead to skin cancer. But honestly, that seems far away and not immediate enough to wear sunscreen for decades on end. I've had those thoughts too. If you're willing to feed into the reckless tendencies of youth, at least wear sunscreen because you're vain and care about your appearance.

Sun spots, hyperpigmentation, and wrinkles are all exacerbated by sun exposure. You should use sunscreen while healing a breakout if you're not a fan of scars. Everyone is susceptible to hyperpigmentation, including people of color. Melanin may be a natural sunblock, but it's also the very culprit behind those dark spots. If you're a beach bum who just can't get enough sun, then wear sunscreen to increase the longevity of those youthful days on the beach. There's really a reason for everyone, whether you have fair skin or dark skin, are uber health conscious, or are just totally self-absorbed, to use sunscreen. The best part is that there are tons of options for both physical sunscreens and chemical sunscreens.

PHYSICAL SUNSCREENS are made up of minerals that act as a physical shield on the skin. Examples include zinc oxide and titanium dioxide. These are some of the most effective sunscreens because they are able to scatter the UV rays that hit the surface of your skin and prevent absorption. The major downside is that some formulations leave a white pasty residue, though this is a category of rapid innovation, with the latest being clear and even tinted sunscreens.

CHEMICAL SUNSCREENS have been a staple for years because of their easy application and much more forgiving appearance on the skin. There are tons of different chemicals used in these formulations, and they work to scavenge free radicals as well as absorb the UV rays directly and release that energy as heat. They protect against UVA and UVB rays and are typically given the designation broad spectrum. A major downside for people with oily or acne-prone skin is that these sunscreens can clog pores and cause breakouts.

Sunscreens come in a variety of application methods, and I'm sure you can find one that fits your lifestyle, like a roll-on stick that looks more like a deodorant and doesn't get all over your hands or make a mess. There are also compact sunscreens that are equal parts chic and equal parts UV protective.

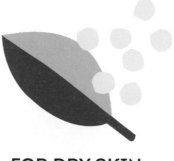

FOR DRY SKIN

The collection of dry skin routines here has two main goals: 1) to prevent excessive drying, and 2) to provide more moisture to your skin. When you're looking for a routine to help you handle the dry patches and flaky skin that seem to persist no matter what time of year, flip through the next few pages to find some salvation.

With dry skin comes the occasional oil streak where your skin is trying to overcompensate for the lack of oil by producing excess sebum. A sudden oily streak isn't a good sign, so you'll want to continue to work on bringing more moisture to the skin while also balancing a potential acne breakout. I know, it's tough.

Then there are those nights when you're all hands on deck and ready to dedicate some real time to your skin. You made the right choice. Let's walk through some intensive treatments to help you reset your skin and get it back on track.

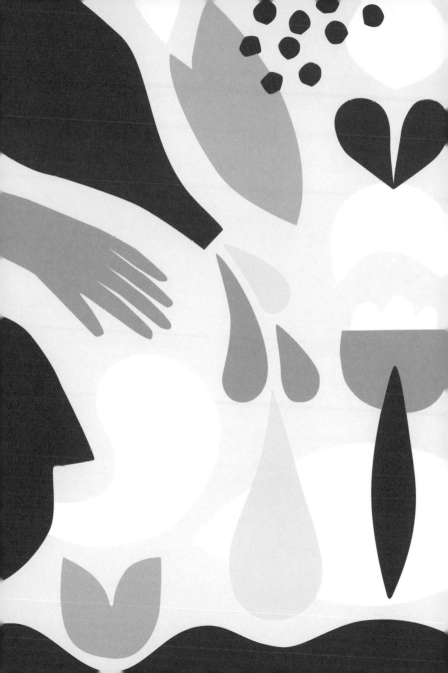

Hydrating Regimen

This is your go-to routine for dry skin. No matter what kind of day you're having, these are the basics you can apply to work toward moisturized, dewy skin.

CLEANSE. Use an oil cleanser to begin. (If you have oily skin, skip this step.)

CLEANSE. Use a water-based cleanser. (If it's wintertime or the weather is especially dry, skip this step.)

EXFOLIATE. You want to remove any dead skin cells from the surface of your face with a salicylic acid exfoliating solution. Gently pat the exfoliant onto your face with both hands, starting with your forehead and moving systematically from the middle out.

APPLY TONER. A toner with sulfur will help remove dead skin, and it's also a great way to begin the acne healing process by drying out a pimple if you're dealing with a breakout. Gently pat the toner onto the surface of your face with two hands, taking care to cover every area. Let your toner dry for a minute before moving on to the next step.

5

APPLY SERUM. A serum with rosehip oil will feel like rubbing the velvety petals of a dozen roses onto your face. You only need a few drops to take advantage of their moisturizing capabilities and drink in that decadent aroma. Flakes may be a symptom of your dry skin, and this step will ensure that you continue to renew your skin as it dries and peels off.

6

MOISTURIZE. Layer on a thick moisturizer to finish up this routine. Look for ingredients like shea, hyaluronic acid, glycerin, aloe vera, and caprylic triglyceride that help lock in moisture by reducing water loss.

AFFIRMATION

I CHOOSE TO NURTURE MYSELF
TODAY AND EVERY DAY.

Crisis Mode: Dry Patches

This is an intensive treatment to remedy your dry patches or bouts of extremely dry skin. Do this in addition to your usual dry skin-care routine. Essentially, we're going to drown your face in incredible hydrating ingredients until it starts to feel better. Yes, there are two masking steps in this routine. The first is a wash-off mask, while the second is what I'm calling a *bask*. You heard it here first. *Basking (v)* is the act of unapologetically living your best life while simultaneously masking to reach your skin goals; often used to describe the process of winding down in bathleisure while masking without regard for others because you don't owe anyone anything. You'll want to light a candle and set the mood because basking is your new best friend.

AFFIRMATION

THIS IS MY DOMAIN: I CAN HANDLE ANYTHING.

1 **HUMIDIFY.** Stand about 6 in (15 cm) away from a humidifier with a towel draped over your head and the steam vent to help channel the steam toward you for 5 minutes. If you don't have a humidifier, you can run a very hot shower and hang out in the steam or lay a steamy washcloth (not too hot!) over your face. Applying steam to your face will begin the hydration process with nature's first beauty ingredient, H2O, and encourage sweat and toxins to move to the surface of your skin.

2 **APPLY MASK.** Use your fingers or a mask brush to evenly apply a bentonite clay mask to your face. Be sure to cover your nose, under-eye area, and neck. This type of mask will reduce inflammation and dry out any pimples you might be dealing with. Leave in place for 10 to 15 minutes, or as directed by the product packaging. To prevent overdrying, don't go beyond the time indicated on your specific mask.

3 **APPLY SECOND MASK.** Use your fingers or a mask brush to evenly apply a hyaluronic acid mask to your face. Be sure to cover your nose, under-eye area, and neck. This type of mask will restore moisture to your face after using a drying clay mask. Leave in place for 10 to 15 minutes, or as directed by the product packaging, whichever is longer. If you are using a sheet mask, simply lay the sheet evenly over your face, making sure to avoid your eyes. Remove when the mask begins to dry out.

4 APPLY SERUM. Apply 3 to 4 drops of tea tree serum to your face. It will soothe your itching and irritation. If you're dealing with a breakout, you can use a tea tree serum as a spot treatment. Be sure to spread it evenly across all the major surfaces on your face.

5 MOISTURIZE. Take a quarter-size dollop of moisturizer into your palm and rub your hands together. Gently work the moisturizer into your face, making sure to cover every surface.

6 HUMIDIFY, ROUND 2. If the air is particularly dry, consider leaving the humidifier on in your bedroom while you sleep.

7 APPLY THIRD MASK (OPTIONAL). If you're interested in creating the perfect addition to that bedhead look, go for an additional sleep mask to lull you into your dreams.

An Oily Streak

When you have dry skin, an oily streak can feel like a blessing, but don't think that's permission to take a day off. One day can be ignored, but when you're on the morning of day 3, it's time to step in and take a closer look. Feel your face for any emerging blemishes, get a sense of the landscape, and take note of any bumps you come across.

CLEANSE. Use a dry cloth to wipe your face and remove excess oils. Rub a teaspoon of coconut oil (or your favorite oil-based cleanser) between your hands and gently work it into your face. Wet your face cloth with warm water and use it to wipe the oil off your face. You can also run a hot shower to steam the room or use your humidifier for an intensified effect.

CLEANSE ROUND 2. Use a water-based cleanser to remove the remaining coconut oil from your face, along with any leftover grime.

APPLY TONER. Use a hydrating toner with hyaluronic acid to bring some moisture back to your face. Gently pat the toner onto your face with both hands, starting with your forehead and moving systematically from the middle out and the top down.

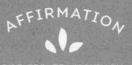

APPLY SERUM (OPTIONAL). Drop 3 drops of a hyaluronic acid serum or your favorite hydrating serum into your palm. Mix with your moisturizer.

MOISTURIZE. Choose a moisturizer with squalane—it's an ingredient that's helpful for regulating oil production while also hydrating the skin. Take a quarter-size amount of moisturizer into your palm and rub your hands together. Gently work the moisturizer into your face, using more as needed, making sure to cover every surface.

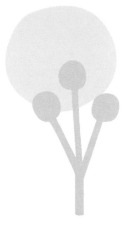

FOR OILY SKIN

Having oil on the skin is a good thing; being dewy is a blessing. But when that goes too far, you've got to rein it back in. These routines will 1) help you deal with day-to-day symptoms, 2) give you a road map for dry patches, and 3) leave you with a little peace of mind.

On the flip side, sometimes oily skin experiences short periods of dryness. That's not a sign of success, but rather of imbalance. So in those cases we'll work on restoring moisture to the skin to bring back that natural glow. That's where an intensive night in comes into play, both for your skin and for a little personal restoration.

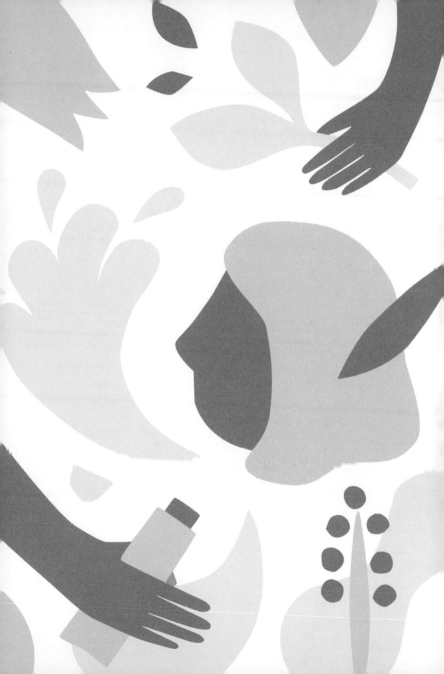

The Mattifying Regimen

This is your go-to routine for managing oily skin. No matter what kind of day you're having, these are the basics you can apply to work toward balanced, happy skin.

CLEANSE. Use a dry cloth to wipe your face and remove excess oils. Then apply a water-based cleanser in a circular motion to work the solution into a lather.

EXFOLIATE. You want to remove any dead skin cells from the surface of your face with either a physical or chemical exfoliator. Gently work through the daily buildup that may accumulate on your skin's surface.

APPLY TONER. A toner that includes bentonite clay will give you that mattified finish that is so elusive when you have oily skin. Gently pat this toner onto your face using both hands.

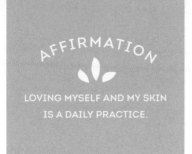

MOISTURIZE. A light moisturizing lotion or cream
will give you an airy finish and will also hydrate you. If
you want to stay matte, forgo an oil-based moisturizer
and stick with a water-based formula. Use about a
nickel-size amount or just enough to lightly cover the full
surface of your skin.

APPLY SUNSCREEN. Always apply sunscreen before
you leave the house. A physical sunscreen with zinc oxide
has a different texture than a chemical sunscreen and
won't leave you feeling oily and sticky in the sun. You can
skip this step by using a moisturizer with SPF.

Crisis Mode: Greasy Skin

Oily skin can be caused by a lot of things, but one of the most common causes is hormone production, particularly for women, as hormone levels change during the menstrual cycle. This can lead to skin feeling greasier at different times during the month. Hormonal acne is also tied to this phenomenon and typically appears along your chin, on your upper lip, and your forehead. But no matter the cause, this routine can help you get a handle on those moments when your oil level feels out of control.

CLEANSE. Use a dry cloth to wipe your face to remove excess oils. Rub a teaspoon of hempseed oil between your hands and gently work it into your face. Wet your face cloth with warm water and use it to wipe the oil off your face. You can also run a hot shower to steam the room or use a humidifier for an intensified effect.

CLEANSE ROUND 2. Use a water-based cleanser to remove the remaining hempseed oil from your face and any leftover grime. A solution with a lactic acid content of 3 percent or less is very hydrating, making it a good ingredient to seek out. Above that threshold you will start to head into exfoliating territory.

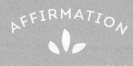

APPLY TONER. Use a hydrating toner with hyaluronic acid to bring some moisture back to your face. Gently pat the toner onto your face with both hands, starting with your forehead and moving systematically from the middle out. Let it dry for 30 seconds and go for a second layer.

APPLY SERUM (OPTIONAL). Drop 3 drops of a hyaluronic acid serum or your favorite hydrating serum into your palm. Mix with your moisturizer.

MOISTURIZE. Choose a moisturizer with squalane. Squalane is helpful for regulating oil production while also hydrating the skin. Take a quarter-size portion into your palm and rub your hands together. Gently work the moisturizer into your face, making sure to cover every surface.

A Dry Spell

Even with oily skin, there are some days when your skin feels
a bit dry and tight. This often happens during the change of a
season or during long air travel. This routine is similar to some
of the dry skin–care routines, but with a few modifications.
This is all about building up your skin barrier and bringing
more moisture to your face.

AFFIRMATION

TODAY I WILL TUNE IN TO MY
OWN FREQUENCY AND DIVE
DEEP INTO MY ENERGY.

HUMIDIFY. Stand about 6 in (15 cm) away from your humidifier with a towel draped over your head for 5 minutes. If you don't have a humidifier you can run a very hot shower or lay a steamy washcloth (not too hot!) over your face. Applying steam to your face will begin the hydration process with nature's first beauty ingredient, H2O, and encourage sweat and toxins to move to the surface of your skin.

CLEANSE. Use a gel cleanser to clean your face. It will be light, soothing, and hydrating to your skin.

APPLY MASK. Use your fingers or a mask brush to evenly apply your favorite hyaluronic acid mask to your face—this ingredient will help moisturize your skin. Be sure to cover your nose, under-eye area, and neck. Leave in place for 10 to 15 minutes, or as directed by the product packaging. If you are using a sheet mask, simply lay the sheet evenly over your face, making sure to avoid your eyes. Remove when the mask begins to dry out.

4 APPLY SERUM. Apply 3 to 4 drops of grape seed oil serum to your face to improve moisture retention. Be sure to spread it evenly across your face.

5 APPLY SECOND MASK. Use your fingers or a mask brush to evenly apply your favorite gel mask to your face. The combination of a lightweight gel, the cooling nature of its formulations, and the hydrating components make it an incredibly soothing mask when your skin is irritated. Be sure to cover your nose, under-eye area, and neck. This type of mask will provide intense rehydration. Rub into face. No need to wash off.

6 MOISTURIZE. Put a quarter-size amount of moisturizer into your palm, and rub your hands together. Gently work the moisturizer into your face, making sure to cover every surface.

7 HUMIDIFY, ROUND 2. If the air is particularly dry, consider leaving the humidifier on in your bedroom while you sleep.

8 APPLY THIRD MASK (OPTIONAL). If you're interested in turning up the dial on that bedhead look, go for an additional sleep mask to lull you into your dreams.

FOR LONGEVITY

First let's address the elephant in the room: anti-aging. This is what some would call the anti-aging section of the book. I don't think there's anything wrong with "signs of aging." I like to think longevity is a blessing. But if one of your goals is to make it harder for people to guess your age, then that's something I can get behind.

Taking care of your skin as you age is as much about taking care of yourself emotionally as physically. Part of how we determine whether or not our skin is healthy is by how beautiful we perceive it to be—and that's okay. Waking up to discover new lines that won't go away with a little rub, or darker circles from several years of missed sleep will take more than a cream to work through. Besides, those aren't signs of unhealthy skin. Those are the marks that come with the wear and tear of living a full life. No one should ever make you self-conscious about laugh lines. Be grateful for that joyful noise. However, aging the way you want to requires that you start early. Regardless of age, you should be thinking about your skin in the long term.

There are two ways in which the skin ages: intrinsically (internal factors) and extrinsically (external factors). Intrinsic aging is the result of the internal aging process that happens for every organ in your body, metabolic processes, and hormone regulation. So even if you stayed indoors for the next 50 years you would still see changes associated with aging creep up on you. But you can slow down the outward appearance of these factors by guarding yourself from excessive sun exposure—the biggest external factor in skin aging. Darker skin will show these signs more slowly, because the melanin that causes the darker skin tone also acts as a natural sunscreen. "Black don't crack" isn't just a stereotype—it's also based in science. But there is a lot you can do if you are not so well endowed in that department.

Sun exposure is the largest contributor, besides time, to wrinkles, spots, scars, and fine lines. So if your focus is to get some sun, then you need to invest in a good sunscreen and retinoid cream. Together these two products will prevent unhealthy skin damage that could lead to cancer and burning while boosting collagen production and skin elasticity.

So here's to longevity. May it suit you, may it favor you, and may you look beautiful always!

Start 'Em Young

In the years leading up to fine lines and sun spots, you can make a real difference in the pace at which your skin shows signs of aging. A large part of that will be incorporating vitamin A into your routine now and for years to come. You'll often see this listed as retinol on the ingredient label, but that's just the name for the vitamin A derivative that is used in skin-care products. It's effective for reducing the appearance of fine lines, spurring collagen production, and increasing cell turnover. Using it early on will improve the longevity of your skin's youthful appearance.

CLEANSE. Apply a gentle cleanser to your face and work into each area by moving your fingers in a circular motion. Start from the center and move outward and top to bottom.

EXFOLIATE. A physical exfoliator twice a week will help to reduce the buildup of dead skin on the surface of your face. The buildup can cause the appearance of aging skin, and thus it's an easy way to "buff" your face.

APPLY TONER. Salicylic acid (SA) toner is the perfect daily exfoliator. SA is a beta hydroxy acid that gently exfoliates and peels. In the form of a toner, you get a relatively mild effect and can use this more often than a typical peel. Follow the packaging for further instructions on proper usage.

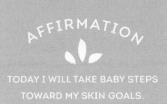

4 APPLY RETINOL. A retinoid cream is best applied at night before going to bed to improve elasticity and the appearance of fine lines and to encourage collagen production, all factors that contribute to the longevity of your skin. You can work it into your skin using the under-eye massage on page 175.

5 MOISTURIZE. A moisturizer with vitamin E or shea will hydrate your skin and encourage longevity. This step cannot be skipped. Increased moisture loss is something we all deal with as we age, making moisturizing an essential part of this routine. Use a quarter-size amount to spread evenly across your face. If you have skin on the dry side, you may want to use more.

6 APPLY SUNSCREEN: If you're headed out the door, finish up with a physical sunscreen that has zinc oxide. Photodamage is one of the largest contributors to the development of wrinkles and sunspots.

Life's a Betch

Life throws a lot at us. That can mean family responsibilities, demanding careers, or extracurricular leadership commitments, all of which leave less time for you and your skin. I bet you've even scaled back your self-care routines to make room for packing school lunches or pushing your career that extra mile. It may also mean years of unprotected sun exposure. Using a peel to reach your longevity goals can be a bit intensive for some skin types. No one should peel more than once a week and if that's too intense, you can reduce the frequency to every other week. Here's a routine for dealing with the photodamage and fine lines that come along with years of vacations and chasing your dreams under the sun.

1 CLEANSE. Apply a gentle cleanser to your face and work into each area by moving three fingers in a circular motion.

2 PEEL. Apply an acid peel that contains polyhydroxy acids to your face once a week to deal with sun spots and scarring, and to resurface the skin for a more even complexion. Depending on how irritated this makes your skin, it's okay to do this every other week.

3 APPLY SERUM. Follow the peel with a soothing tea tree oil. It will reduce the inflammation and irritation that may result from an abrasive peel. Its antiseptic properties will also be a huge benefit to preventing any side effects. It also doubles as a great spot treatment for adult acne.

4 APPLY RETINOL. Apply a retinoid containing cream or emulsion to your face. This step is important and will focus on collagen production, cell renewal, and reducing the appearance of fine lines.

5 MOISTURIZE. In the context of aging and longevity, hydrating your skin is very important because it tends to more or less "retire" its own hydrating function as we get older.

6 APPLY SUNSCREEN. If you're headed out the door, finish up with a physical sunscreen that has zinc oxide. Photodamage is one of the largest contributors to the development of wrinkles and sunspots, and it's never too late to start protecting your skin.

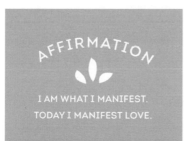

AFFIRMATION

I AM WHAT I MANIFEST.
TODAY I MANIFEST LOVE.

Stuck in Crow Pose

Crow's-feet are a tell-tale sign of years spent squinting into the future. Now you're here and you're probably wondering how to make them go away. Under-eye creams are incredibly popular in the "anti-aging" section of the beauty department. The fact is that the skin under and around your eyelids, while a bit thinner, is essentially the same as that around your face. You don't have to purchase separate products for your eyes, because a general retinol will be just as effective. This routine can also be supplemented with an eye-centric face massage that you can find on page 175. Do it after the moisturizing step and before the sleep mask.

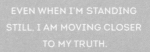

AFFIRMATION

EVEN WHEN I'M STANDING
STILL, I AM MOVING CLOSER
TO MY TRUTH.

1 **CLEANSE.** Apply a gentle cleanser to your face and work it into each area by moving three fingers in a circular motion starting from the middle and moving outward.

2 **EXFOLIATE.** A physical exfoliator twice a week will help to reduce the buildup of dead skin on the surface of your face. The buildup can cause the appearance of aging skin, and thus it's an easy way to "buff" your face.

3 **APPLY TONER.** Salicylic acid toner is the perfect daily exfoliator for dealing with sun spots and scars. SA is a betahydroxy acid that gently exfoliates and peels. In the form of a toner, you get a relatively mild effect and can use this more often than a typical peel. Follow the packaging for further instructions on proper usage.

4 **APPLY MASK.** A regenerating mask with AHAs, BHAs, and vitamin A work to regenerate the skin and peel back layers of dead cells. This is also a bit intensive, so don't skip the soothing moisturizing step that follows.

5 APPLY RETINOL. Apply a retinoid-containing cream or emulsion to your face. This step is important and will focus on collagen production, cell renewal, and reducing the appearance of fine lines.

6 MOISTURIZE. In the context of aging, hydrating your skin is very important because our skin tends to more or less "retire" this function as we get older. The creases and lines tend to appear in areas where plumping moisture has begun to decrease.

7 MASSAGE YOUR EYES. Exercise the muscles around your eyes with the invigorating massage on page 175. This will bring more circulation to the area as well.

8 APPLY A SLEEP MASK. A hydrating sleep mask will keep your face nice and plump throughout the night. A lot of water loss happens as you sleep, which is why many people wake up feeling dehydrated. Have a glass of water before you settle into bed.

TO REFLECT
HOW YOU EAT

Your skin is equally a reflection of the internal state of your body and the lifestyle choices you make to take care of it. Incorporating your dietary choices into your skin-care routine is an incredible holistic way to approach the process of self-care. If you choose to eat a plant-based diet, apply those same principles to your skin-care routine. If probiotics are part of your gut health journey, there's no reason why they can't be part of your skin-care journey as well. Taking care of your body is about seeking balance. The gut-skin-brain axis is the communication channel between your psyche, your gut microbiome, and your skin flora, and their health is all connected. In the next few routines we'll cover specific microbiome-safe products to use, and how to bring your plant-based diet into the bathroom.

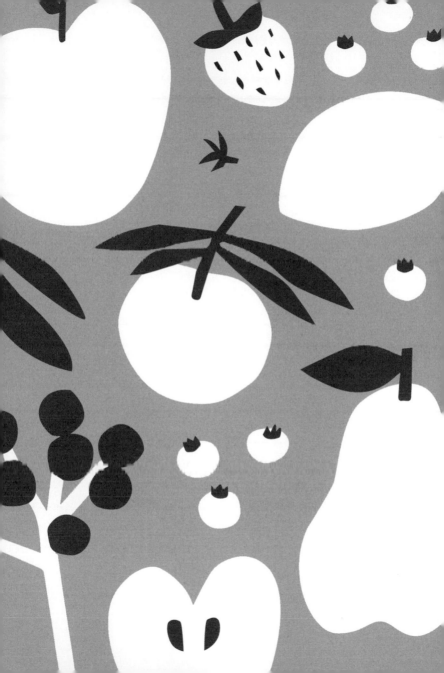

Survival of the Fittest

Part of maintaining a healthy and balanced skin microbiome is avoiding the ingredients and external factors that can cause it to get out of whack. For instance, using broad-spectrum antimicrobials or antibacterial products will indiscriminately rid your skin of all kinds of bacteria, even if they are beneficial to the skin. Common skin-care ingredients like essential oils have powerful antibacterial qualities. So though they may smell very nice, if your focus is on cultivating your skin's natural ecosystem, avoid essential oils because they are not very microbiome friendly. Linoleic oils like poppy seed, grape seed, sunflower, hemp, and coconut can stay on your nice list. Most essential oils should be used in moderation. This is a less-is-more routine. As it turns out, low-maintenance skin care is one of the best ways to let your skin do its thing.

CLEANSE. Cleanse using a probiotic cleanser with ammonia oxidizing bacteria. These types of bacteria were previously found to be dominant on the skin, but we lost them as we evolved into hyperclean beings. This will bring you back to a purer time, the good old days. These bacteria have been shown to improve moisture, itchiness, dry skin, and acne.

MOISTURIZE. A moisturizer that contains oats, a natural prebiotic, will improve your skin's pH and barrier function and help moisturize your skin and create a friendly environment for those long lost bacteria to thrive. This prebiotic is particularly effective if you have dry skin.

APPLY MASK (OPTIONAL). Use a probiotic sheet mask with *lactobacillus* and *bifidobacterium* if you have more time on your hands. These are friendly bacteria, typically found in your gut, that have been shown to be very good for rebalancing your skin's flora. Yep, that's it.

Muddy Waters

If you're ready to go all in with an extended microbiome friendly routine, this is it. Focusing on your microbiome doesn't mean you have to sacrifice the fun of all the other steps in a routine like, for instance, masking. Once you've gotten the hang of introducing balance into your daily self-care routine, you can begin to add more steps. Let's go a little deeper and get a little dirtier with this muddy routine.

CLEANSE. Cleanse using a probiotic cleanser with ammonia oxidizing bacteria. These types of bacteria were previously found to be dominant on the skin, but we lost them as we evolved into hyperclean beings. This will bring you back to a purer time, the good old days. These bacteria have been known to improve moisture, itchiness, dry skin, and acne.

MASK. Apply a charcoal mask to your face with your hands or a mask brush. Activated charcoal has been shown to primarily fight against *E. coli* and *Staphylococcus aureus* and is relatively microbiome safe.

3

APPLY TONER. Lactic acid toner will reduce the pH of your skin and create the perfect environment for your microbiome to thrive. *Lactobacillus*, which is found in your gut, produces this acid naturally.

4

MOISTURIZE. Kefir is a natural probiotic, similar to yogurt. It has strong moisturizing properties in addition to being able to balance your microbiome and build a better skin barrier. Use a quarter-size amount of a kefir-containing moisturizer to spread evenly across your face.

5

MIST. To finish with a dewy look, spritz your face 2 to 3 times with a symbiotic mist. A symbiotic has both prebiotics and probiotics that work together to balance your skin microbiome. Mists that include beta-glucan and *bifidobacteria* in their ingredients will protect sensitive skin from irritation caused by harsh weather or harsh chemical products.

6

APPLY SUNSCREEN before you leave the house!

AFFIRMATION

SEEING CLEARLY MEANS
LOOKING WITH MY HEART.

Herbivores' Delight

There were no animals harmed in the making of this routine. The use of botanical extracts to achieve skin goals has been in practice for thousands of years. And like many of the first medicines and elixirs, humans continue to look to nature and its fruits to cure ailments, both physical and spiritual. This routine is all about looking to natural ingredients that grow on trees and spring up from the ground.

AFFIRMATION

I AM A CAGE-FREE GODDESS.
I EMBODY A GRASS-FED,
FREE-RANGE, WILD-CAUGHT
KIND OF BEAUTY.

1 CLEANSE. Apply a gentle cleanser to your face and work into each area by moving three fingers in a circular motion. Look for an aloe vera cleanser to also soothe and calm the skin during this first step.

2 APPLY TONER. Apply a grape seed oil toner to the skin. Gently pat the solution with both hands. It has a cornucopia of benefits including wrinkle defense, acne protection, skin moisturizing, and dark-circle fighting.

3 APPLY SERUM. Apply 3 to 4 drops of a rosehip seed oil serum for skin barrier restoration. It is full of vitamin A, which is an important ingredient for skin longevity.

4 MOISTURIZE. A shea-based moisturizing lotion or balm will effectively lock in moisture and condition the skin. It is particularly good at nourishing and restoring the skin's natural barrier.

Get Back to Nature

After some hard work in your garden flexing your green thumb, it's time to decompress and mask in your vegetative paradise. Taking cues from your environment, let's explore a routine that's on the messy side of the tracks. Your hands have been immersed in the soil your plants need to thrive; a clay-based mask will prolong those "of the earth" vibes and mattify your skin after all the sweat that was surely dripping down your face. Keep it simple. All plants need to thrive is good soil, sun, and water—let's take the same approach with your face.

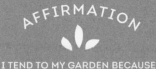

1 **RINSE.** Splash some cold water on your face for a refresh. This will begin your cool-down process and remove some of the salts on your face. A cool, wet towel will also do the trick.

2 **CLEANSE.** Use a water-based cleanser to remove the extra layer of sweat that has accumulated on your skin. Take your time and really work circles around your face. Create as much lather as you can before rinsing off. Lightly pat with a towel.

3 **APPLY MASK.** Use the DIY bentonite clay mask on page 184.

4 **MOISTURIZE.** Use a parsley-seed-containing moisturizing cream. It's high in antioxidants and vitamin C and will be the perfect garden-inspired ingredient to finish off your routine.

FOR ON THE GO

In a tea house in Seoul, South Korea, a guest a few pillows over was curling her bangs while her tea was steeping. Yes, she had a single-battery-powered curling rod that, within 2 minutes, brought new bounce to her brow-grazing tendrils. It showed me that even while on the go, you can do little things for yourself that make you feel and look better. A little extra preparation is all you need.

When we travel, we're forced to fit our beauty routine into 3.4-oz units and resealable bags, and then lock them away until we arrive at our destination. Makeup holds privileged real estate in our purses and backpacks, but rarely do we leave room for our skin-care products. However, your skin goes through so much when you're in transit. It would be nice if all our skin-care needs could be taken care of in the comfort of our bathrooms and bedrooms, but sometimes you need to handle what life throws at you while you're on the move.

Being prepared is the first step, and that includes having a special mini self-care pack in your purse or backpack at all times. It also might mean moving your routine to an airport bathroom as you exfoliate before a flight. Who doesn't want to be that person who has it together enough to mask on the train to visit Grandma?

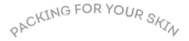

Here is a quick guide to packing the essentials for each skin type when traveling. Travel-size packs are an easy way to bring what you need, wherever you're going. They are also an opportunity to think about the bare bones of your skin-care routine and which products are the most essential.

Choose a 3- or 5-step routine. Packing a combination product helps reduce the number of bottles in your luggage. Go for a combo toner and exfoliator, or exfoliating cleanser. A sheet mask can be tucked in your luggage. Remember to check the weather at your destination, as you'll want to coordinate your skin care with your outfits.

Keep a separate toilet bag dedicated only to your travel skin-care routine. You can pour your favorite products into small plastic bottles you find at the drugstore, or simply purchase the travel sizes of each product. In short, there's no reason why you can't take care of your skin while you're getting some much needed R and R.

PACKING FOR 1 WEEK OR LONGER

If you could travel with your full at-home setup, I'm sure you would. But a few weeks is not enough time to warrant many large suitcases. However, it is just the right amount of time for a surprise skin concern.

Cleanser: cleansing wipes or a travel-size cleanser
Toner/Exfoliator: a combination exfoliating toner paired with exfoliating cotton pads, so you don't skip a beat
Serum: tea tree oil (this doubles as a spot treatment, a moisturizer, and an anti-inflammatory ingredient)
Moisturizer: travel-size moisturizer
Mask: 2–3 sheet masks, or a tube of your favorite mask

PACKING FOR THE WEEKEND

Cleanser: cleansing wipes
Toner: combination toner/emulsion
Moisturizer: travel-size moisturizer
Mask: sheet mask that you can use in transit or at your destination

ON-THE-GO STAPLES

Facial mist spray
Moisturizing face lotion
Exfoliating sponge

The Freshen Up (No Makeup)

There's that moment during the day when you've been walking around getting stuff done, and then you catch a glimpse of yourself. Oh no. Why didn't anyone tell you that you had a fresh zit, a persistent layer of sweat and, is that . . . ketchup or red marker on your chin? This routine is for one of those days.

AFFIRMATION

A REFRESHED SPIRIT IS A
BRAND-NEW BEGINNING.

USE A CLEANSING WIPE. Break out that stash of cleansing wipes from your go pack (see page 109) and begin to wipe in long even strokes, starting from the bottom of your chin and moving upward.

APPLY TONER. Splash some toner onto your cleansing wipe, and apply it in upward strokes across your face. Ideally this is either an exfoliating toner or a hydrating toner. Either will give your face a renewed glow.

MOISTURIZE. You don't need to overdo this. Just a light once-over with your favorite travel moisturizer will be more than enough.

MIST. Before you walk out of the bathroom or broom closet you slid into, give your face one refreshing spritz. You'll look dewy, like you just emerged from a saucy afternoon delight.

FIND A MESSAGE IN A BOTTLE: For a quick 15-second reset, go for a mist. They are lightweight, smell good, and add a little luxury to your day. It's the closest to bottling therapy and meditation that the skin-care industry has come. Mists are making it possible to tone on the subway or refresh moisture levels in between meetings. Most mists will work even if you have makeup on.

The Freshen Up (Makeup)

Sometimes long-lasting makeup doesn't really make it to the end of the day—to say nothing of the skin underneath it. Here's a quick way to freshen your face that will only mildly mess up your makeup. Taking a moment to do a little touch-up can get you through the final stretch.

USE A CLEANSING WIPE. Break out that stash of cleansing wipes from your go pack (see page 109) and begin to wipe in short strokes only over the areas of concern. You can fold your wipe into triangles for more precision.

SPOT TREAT. There are three options for spot treating:
- clay mask for a current or emerging pimple
- exfoliating lotion for any grime that's parked on your face
- hydrating toner for skin that's feeling very dry.

Dab one or more of these products onto the problem area and then clean off with your cleansing wipe.

EXFOLIATE with a dry to damp exfoliating brush. A charcoal exfoliating brush is easy to pack, won't cause any redness or irritation, and will quickly rejuvenate your face. Use only on problem spots if you want to preserve your makeup.

MOISTURIZE. Dab moisturizer onto that fresh skin, and reapply your makeup as needed.

Late for Your 3 O'Clock

Have you ever tried to just escape your day like a kid running away from home to join the circus? Where do you go when you try to escape? What do you do when you can't? I often feel this way when I'm running in between meetings, or when I remember that I still haven't replied to that "urgent" email from a colleague. I break out my lotion or face mist for a minute reprieve. The smell of almond, coconut, and bitter orange immediately transports me, and I don't have to take a step. Sometimes I add a brief meditation to lock in the experience.

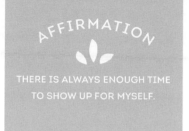

1   **BREATHE.** Close your eyes. Take a deep breath in and hold it for 3 counts, release for 3 counts. Repeat 3 times.

 MIST. Choose your favorite calming mist spray. I would recommend a rosewater facial mist. Close your eyes and pump 3 spritzes onto your face. Other ingredients to seek out: patchouli, tangerine, chamomile, tea tree oil, coconut.

3   **DO A MEDITATION MANTRA.** Take 3 minutes to close your eyes and slow down your breathing. When you've reached a comfortable position, repeat these words: This is my time. This is my space.

Going Upstate for the Holidays

With a few hours on the train, you can leisurely work on your glow to impress even your cool cousins. With a little spare time in between leaving the office and eating your mom's corn bread, you can create a little sanctuary for yourself on the trip. When you're 30 minutes from your final destination, break out a sheet mask and do a little face massage to help you face your family. The holidays are all about spreading love; there's no reason why you can't shower it on yourself.

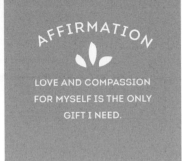

1 **USE A CLEANSING WIPE.** Take off the stress from the day. Use a wipe to gently remove any makeup or sweat that may be on your face.

2 **APPLY A SHEET MASK.** Use a calming sheet mask that contains ceramides and licorice root to hydrate your face. Lay the sheet mask evenly across your face and leave it on for 10 to 15 minutes.

3 **MASSAGE.** Give yourself a quick reboot with a face massage. See the Facial Massages section on page 173 for a few options that will circulate the blood in your face and reduce any puffiness you may have.

4 **MIST.** Using your favorite mist, spritz 2 to 3 times and pat the mist into your face using both hands. The refreshed, dewy glow will give you that holiday sparkle you've been chasing.

When You're on a 14-Hour Flight

You made it through that crazy security line. Now what? Head to the bathroom to do a little preflight cleansing/moisturizing/etc. An airplane cabin is dryer than the Sahara Desert, so the routine continues with a relaxing in-flight mask. If you're worried about looking crazy, don't. Those in the know will be impressed with the fact that you thought about your skin on this trip. You're an advanced traveler now. Welcome to the club.

This routine focuses on moisturizing every step of the way. Hyaluronic acid is a key ingredient because it naturally attracts water, and you're gonna need it for this transcontinental journey.

AFFIRMATION

TODAY I WILL CONNECT TO THE UNIVERSE AROUND ME.

Slip into the airport bathroom:

CLEANSE. Pull out your cleansing wipes. We need to wash off that TSA stress sweat. Remove any makeup you may be wearing, and let your skin breathe a little.

EXFOLIATE. Lightly exfoliate with an exfoliating sponge. This step will help get any residue from sweat and makeup off your face and remove any dead cells that may be loose.

APPLY SERUM. Apply 3 to 4 drops of hyaluronic acid serum to form a thin layer over your face. An airplane cabin is extremely dry. After a quick exfoliation, this serum will more easily soak right into your skin.

APPLY A HEAVY MOISTURIZER AND LIP BALM. You want to lock in as much moisture as possible and let very little water escape mid-flight. A heavy moisturizer will do just the trick. Even if you have oily skin, you don't have to worry; your skin will be begging for water. Slather on a lip balm with beeswax and jojoba oil. Your lips have skin too, and they can get dry and cracked just like any other part of your body during a long flight.

Hop on the plane:

MASK. Buckle up and place a sheet mask on your face. Masks are easy to carry and don't have to be washed off. Let it sit on your face for 15 minutes and then rub in the rest of the emulsion into your skin. It may look awkward, but it will feel great.

Before you land:

CLEANSE AND MOISTURIZE ONE MORE TIME. Use a quick cleansing wipe and more moisturizer; you've lost a lot of moisture while you've been in the air. This will give you that enviable glow as you step off the plane and into your next adventure.

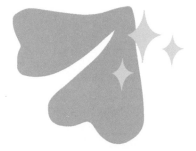

FOR ACNE

Handling a breakout is a fine art, so get ready to pick up your paintbrush. Like any good Picasso, beauty doesn't just appear on a canvas. It takes layers of paint and a few sittings. The first step to dealing with a breakout is to handle the inflammatory response that comes along with it, getting that bump to be as small as possible. Then you'll work on scar prevention so you don't have to live with the aftermath. And for more help on dealing with acne scars, check out routines for hyperpigmentation (page 138).

Fifty-four percent of adults 20 to 40 have some sort of acne, so really, you are not alone in this struggle. Mouth, chin, jawline, neck, and chest are areas where most adults experience breakouts, and that's a reflection of the "adulting" lifestyle. Factors like stress, pollution, and poor diet cause acne in adults to be more inflammatory. So not only are we dealing with acne later in life, but also skin with different tendencies than our teenage selves were used to. Let's talk about what to do when you have a breakout.

HOW DO PIMPLES WORK?

A pimple starts with hyperkeratosis (thickening) of the skin around the hair follicle. Then an excess of sebum piles up, suffocating the follicle and depriving it of oxygen such that the acne bacteria that are there begin to multiply. This causes inflammation and a small change in your gut microbiome. Add on lifestyle behaviors that increase the presence of acne, like skipping your evening cleanse, and you increase the severity of the acne flare-up. Voilà! You've got a breakout on your hands.

But if you know the pimple playbook, you can use it to your advantage. When you notice your skin getting too oily, you can use The Mattifying Regimen on page 80 to clean things up. On the other hand, if you're starting to see a little mound form, you know something's brewing, so go for an anti-inflammatory ingredient like tea tree oil to calm things down. Being armed with the knowledge of this process will allow you to handle breakouts in a healthy way.

Surprise!

One day you wake up from your beauty sleep and look in the mirror, expecting to see your usual glowing goddess, only to find the latest bad boy has parked right on your face. Try not to freak out. What we commonly refer to as pimples and blemishes are actually the signs that your skin and body use to communicate with you. They're begging for your attention, and it's important that you listen to what they have to say. This is a reminder from your skin that you need to take some downtime for yourself in the midst of all the obligations and stress on your plate. This breakout may be caused by a buildup of dirt because you've been negligent in your skin-care routine. Or maybe your face is asking you to drop that cult-favorite product you just started using because, despite the hype, it's really not gelling with your needs. Here's how to deal with a new breakout.

1

CLEANSE. You'll want to select a nice, gentle foaming cleanser for this one because you really want to work your way around your face. And you'll want it to be water based. You've already got an overproduction of sebum, so less oil is better. Try to avoid an explicitly antimicrobial cleanser because, as you now know, creating an imbalance in the bacteria on the face will only make things worse.

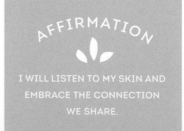

AFFIRMATION

I WILL LISTEN TO MY SKIN AND
EMBRACE THE CONNECTION
WE SHARE.

2 **MASK.** Choose a soothing clay mask with charcoal or sandalwood. Apply all over your face with a second layer on top of any problem areas. You may be stressed because of something going on in your life, or just because you have a new breakout. A calming clay mask will help you relax and dry up that blemish so it is less inflamed and smaller in size.

3 **APPLY TONER.** A calming and anti-inflammatory toner will start to reduce the size of the pimple as well as soothe any painful symptoms it may cause. Choose one with cucumber to really soothe your skin. Use a cotton pad to gently dab the toner directly onto your pimples and around your face. Short strokes in an upward motion increase absorption.

4 **APPLY SERUM.** A salicylic acid or glycolic acid serum is the Holy Grail of blemish-care serums. They work to reduce redness and prevent new breakouts from occurring.

5 **MOISTURIZE.** After a very drying mask, you'll want to restore moisture to your face with a soothing cream. Aloe vera, vitamin E, and chamomile are great ingredients to look out for when managing acne breakouts.

6 **APPLY SUNSCREEN** before you leave the house!

The Morning After

The second day of blemish bliss has a dual focus: more inflammation reduction with a splash of scar prevention. We're still trying to get that blemish down to a size we feel good about, obviously without picking at it or trying to pop that sucker. Trust me, you want to hold back that urge. If you can't stand the sight of this pimple, you certainly won't want to be reminded of it every day with a nasty scar. SPF protection will be crucial to the recovery process too. The sun will exacerbate any scarring or hyperpigmentation that occurs as a result of this blemish. So if you want to truly heal after a breakout, sunscreen has to be part of the solution.

CLEANSE. You'll want to select a nice, gentle foaming cleanser for this one because you really want to work your way around your face. And you'll want it to be water based. You've already got an overproduction of sebum, so less oil is better. Try to avoid an explicitly antimicrobial cleanser because, as you now know, creating an imbalance in the bacteria on the face will only make things worse.

APPLY TONER. An exfoliating toner will begin the process of removing any dead cells from the surface of the pimple. If your pimple is feeling very tender, you can revert to the toner from the routine on page 125 to continue to soothe the area. Exfoliating should not feel painful. If it does, you may be causing more damage to the area.

3

SPOT TREAT. Apply a spot treating solution to the affected areas. You can even use your clay mask as a spot treatment or opt for a solution that contains sulfur.

APPLY SERUM. A salicylic acid or glycolic acid serum is the Holy Grail of blemish-care serums. They work to reduce redness and prevent new breakouts from occurring.

MOISTURIZE. You'll want to restore moisture to your face after all that cleansing with a soothing cream. Aloe vera, vitamin E, and chamomile are great ingredients to look out for when managing acne breakouts.

6

APPLY SUNSCREEN before you leave the house!

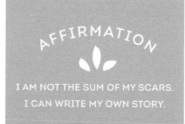

AFFIRMATION

I AM NOT THE SUM OF MY SCARS.
I CAN WRITE MY OWN STORY.

Kale Me Now

Acne is a tricky biospecific condition to manage, and I know how frustrating it can get when you're trying a lot of different products that aren't working. Maybe you've decided that you want to go all botanical and chemical-free with your skin care as a new approach. That's a great idea. For years the prevailing theory was that we needed chemicals to fix our skin, but there are so many natural ingredients that are incredibly effective actives. You shouldn't feel limited by your clean beauty, green beauty lifestyle because there is a lot out there and plenty more to come. For acne management, this routine will take you through several steps and techniques. Feel free to take your own spin on this and leave out what you don't have time for.

AFFIRMATION

I CHOOSE TO EMBODY THE
BEAUTY IN THE NATURAL
ENERGIES THAT FEED ME.

1 **CLEANSE.** Use a dry cloth to wipe your face to remove excess oils. Rub a teaspoon of coconut oil between your hands and gently work it into your skin. Wet your face cloth with warm water and use it to wipe the oil off your face. Run a hot shower to steam the room for an intensified effect.

2 **CLEANSE ROUND 2.** Use a water-based cleanser to remove the remaining coconut oil and any leftover grime from your face. Choose a product with seaweed or algae (sometimes labeled as astaxanthin), both of which have been shown to prevent acne and reduce redness and irritation.

3 **APPLY TONER.** Use a hydrating toner with hyaluronic acid to bring some moisture back to your face. Gently pat the toner onto your face with both hands, starting with your forehead and moving systematically from the middle out and top down. Let it dry for 30 seconds and go for a second layer.

EXFOLIATE. A pumpkin enzyme exfoliating mask will work to resurface your skin and fight against hyperpigmentation. Leave on as instructed. Use a physical exfoliating brush to wash it off for a little extra action.

APPLY SERUM. A salicylic acid or glycolic acid serum is the Holy Grail of blemish-care serums. They work to reduce redness and prevent new breakouts from occurring.

APPLY SERUM, ROUND 2. Apply 3 to 4 drops of a rosehip seed oil serum for skin barrier restoration. It is full of vitamin A, which is an important ingredient for skin longevity. This step tackles acne prevention and longevity in one.

MOISTURIZE. Choose a moisturizer for a light finish, and look for one with parsley seed oil for an antioxidant boost. Take a quarter-size amount of moisturizer into your palm and rub your hands together. Gently work the moisturizer into your face, making sure to cover every surface.

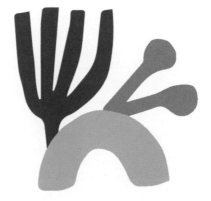

FOR IRRITATED SKIN

Post-Workout Sweat

You showed up for yourself today and went to the gym to get in a good sweat. Now it's time to get out in the world, but not before a little refresher. Step into the locker room and give your face a little skin-care workout. You don't want the sweat to stay on your face all day. The excess oils could lead to a breakout, and honestly, can just feel a little gross. This routine is a quick way to refresh your face after going the extra mile.

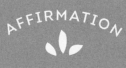

AFFIRMATION

I CHOOSE TO SHOW UP FOR
MYSELF TODAY TO GIVE MY
BODY WHAT IT NEEDS.

1 **RINSE.** Splash some cold water on your face for a refresh. This will begin your cool-down process and remove some of the salts from your face. A cool, wet towel will also do the trick.

2 **CLEANSE.** Use a water-based cleanser to remove the extra layer of sweat that has accumulated on your face from your workout. Take your time and really work circles around your face. Create as much lather as you can before rinsing off. Lightly pat with a towel.

3 **APPLY TONER.** Use a hydrating toner with hyaluronic acid to bring some moisture back to your face after the thorough washing. Gently pat the toner onto your face with both hands, starting with your forehead and moving systematically from the middle out and top down. Let it dry for 1 minute before moving on to the next step.

4 **MOISTURIZE.** Choose a light moisturizer to soothe and moisturize your face. Your body may still be a bit warm from exercising and produce more sweat, so no need to pack on the creams.

5 **MIST.** Spray a gentle rosehip oil mist to close out your glorious workout, a little bit of bliss after all that hard work. Werk it!

Rosacea with Botanical Extracts

The benefit of a vegetarian skin-care routine is that if you focus on natural botanical actives, your skin will benefit from the immense rejuvenating power of plant extracts. From rosehip oil to tea tree oil to shea butter, there are hundreds of thousands of plants and herbs out there that have been used to heal wounds and ailments for centuries. Here's how to unlock nature's bounty for those of you who were gifted a gorgeous rosy complexion.

1 CLEANSE. Use a dry cloth to wipe your face and remove excess oils. Rub a teaspoon of jojoba seed oil or sesame oil between your hands, and gently work it into your face. Wet your face cloth with warm water, and use it to wipe the oil off your skin. You can also run a hot shower to steam the room or use a humidifier for an intensified effect.

2 CLEANSE ROUND 2. Use a water-based cleanser to remove the remaining oil and any leftover grime from your face.

3

APPLY TONER. Use a hydrating toner with hyaluronic acid and chamomile to bring some moisture back to your face as well as reduce redness and inflammation. Gently pat the toner onto your face with both hands, starting with your forehead and moving systematically from the middle out. Let it dry for 30 seconds and go for a second layer.

4

APPLY SERUM. Apply 3 drops of a pomegranate seed serum, which is both a powerful antioxidant and an anti-inflammatory, to your palm. Spread evenly across your face.

5

MOISTURIZE. Choose a moisturizer with kanuka honey. This honey, hailing all the way from New Zealand, has been shown to improve rosacea symptoms and leave you feeling like a snack! Take a quarter-size amount of moisturizer into your palm and rub your hands together. Gently work the moisturizer into your face, making sure to cover every surface.

AFFIRMATION

TODAY I CHOOSE TO SEE THE
SUNRISE IN MY CHEEKS.

FOR HYPERPIGMENTATION

We all know where dark spots come from: the devil. Kidding! But I know I'm not too far off in some of your minds. Part of why we don't love getting pimples is because long after they're gone, we're still contending with the leftovers. *Hyperpigmentation*, or acne scarring, is a huge perpetrator of post-acne embarrassment and frustration. Once you get an acne scar, it can take up to six months for it to make an exit, which means that for the next two fiscal quarters, you're going to be experiencing a boom-bust emotional cycle trying to get over it.

Slow down. What is hyperpigmentation? Good question. It is the discoloration or localized darkening of the skin resulting from overactive *melanocytes*—the cells that produce skin pigment. If you think of a tattoo as ink that lives just below the surface of your skin, your skin is a window and the ink is on the other side of it. Hyperpigmentation is very similar. Melanocytes produce so much pigment that the pigment falls beneath the surface of the skin to lower levels, where it resides. Because those layers are farther down, these spots tend to stick around for longer than some of us would like. And hyperpigmentation is not just caused by acne—it can also appear as age spots related to years of tanning or during pregnancy due to a shift in hormones.

The best way to deal with hyperpigmentation is to focus on some of your bad habits, like not wearing sunscreen. The UV rays from the sun are responsible for exacerbating the appearance of a dark spot. Similarly, when you dry freshly manicured nails under a fan and UV lamp, the light from the lamp hardens the polish and brightens the color to help the manicure look vibrant all week long. So if you expose your skin to sun without the power of protective SPF, you're actually extending the life of that dark spot by concentrating its pigment. By exfoliating and using sunblock, you can improve the appearance of your hyperpigmentation and prevent more of it in the future.

Scrub-a-Dub
(Chemical Exfoliate)

Using a chemical exfoliator, also known as a peel, is one way to work toward a more even complexion. These are typically solutions you apply to your face that dislodge the top layers of your skin by interrupting cell-to-cell bonds. You don't have to scrub to get these off; it's all in the chemistry. A chemical peel should not be incorporated into your routine more than once a week, as it is very abrasive to the skin—on purpose—and can cause damage if done excessively. But in moderation, it can do wonders for removing hyperpigmentation and evening out your skin tone.

APPLY EXFOLIATING CLEANSER. Typically these contain a physical element, like coffee grounds or sugar, that works to resurface the skin while leaving you feeling invigorated.

APPLY TONER. An exfoliating toner is a great addition on most days, and especially when you're working toward a more even skin tone. It's important to apply the toner in staccato upward strokes, starting from your chin and making your way up. Rinse as directed.

PEEL. You'll want to follow the instructions on the packaging of the product to safely extract the most superficial layer of your skin. Be sure that you're timing this step because keeping on a chemical peel for longer than directed can make the peel work a little *too* well.

4

APPLY SERUM. Patchouli oil is an intense healing essential oil that will soothe your skin after using an astringent peel. It will also soothe any inflammation in response to the peel as well as provide the antiseptic protection you'll need from exposing new layers of your skin.

5

MOISTURIZE. Use a moisturizer that contains soy or a soy derivative. Soy has been found to prevent the transfer of pigment to the surface of the skin while also lightening its appearance.

6

APPLY SUNSCREEN before you leave the house! Sun damage can make hyperpigmentation look worse, so it's doubly important to protect your skin from harmful rays.

Let's Get Physical, Physical (Physical Exfoliation)

Physical exfoliation is one of the safest ways to remove dead skin, grime, and debris from your face. It's worth doing not just on your face, but also on your neck and décolletage. Those are all areas where you can get buildup from sweat, pollution, and daily wear and tear. Do this up to twice a week to keep your face looking fresh.

APPLY EXFOLIATING CLEANSER. Typically these contain a physical element, like a microbead or a sugar, that works to physically dislodge the dead cells from the top layer of your skin.

APPLY TONER. An exfoliating toner is a great addition on most days, and especially when you're working toward a more even skin tone. It's important to apply the toner in staccato upward strokes, starting from your chin and making your way up. Rinse as directed.

EXFOLIATE. Use a sugar-based scrub to lift dead skin from the surface of your face for a second round of exfoliation. Gently work your way around your face in tight circles. You can do this with an exfoliating sponge for maximum effect.

APPLY MASK (OPTIONAL). A niacinamide mask will improve the appearance of uneven skin tone that may result from a breakout. It will give you that even skin glow you're searching for.

APPLY SERUM. Choose a serum of your liking. You've just removed a layer of dead skin, so this is an opportunity to indulge in nutrients that you feel you may need right at the newest surface of your skin.

MOISTURIZE. Use a moisturizer that contains persimmon, a fruit native to Korea, China, and Japan, which has vitamin A, vitamin E, and carotene. This nutrient can be used to improve the evenness of your skin tone and prevent signs of aging, like fine lines and wrinkles.

APPLY SUNSCREEN before you leave the house!

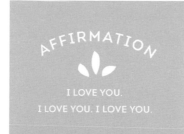

AFFIRMATION

I LOVE YOU.
I LOVE YOU. I LOVE YOU.

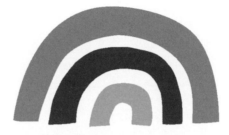

FOR WHEN YOU
NEED A PICK-ME-UP

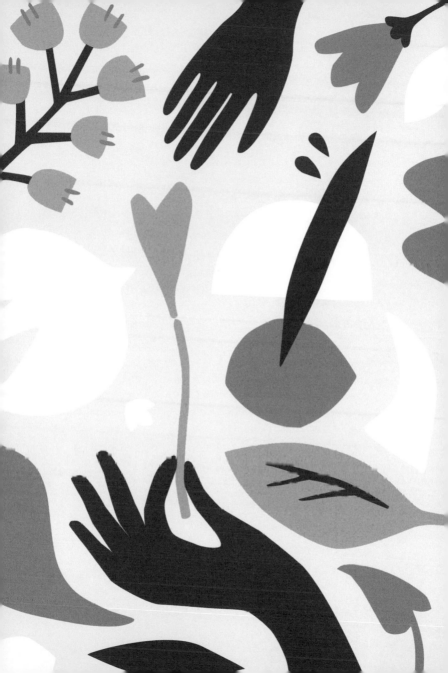

I'll Take My Latte To Go

We've all had those mornings where we snoozed three times too many, or we just couldn't seem to get out of bed. You've probably calculated the last possible second you need to throw on a fresh shirt before your boss will notice how late you are.

You've got 10 minutes before you'll officially be 15 minutes late. Let's make use of that crunch time to handle the bare essentials before you leave the house. This routine is all about getting right to the point without any fluff. If you're still reading this, you've got 9 minutes . . .

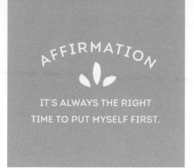

1 **CLEANSE.** Use a facial cleansing wipe to clean your face while you brush your teeth. You can do this with one hand!

2 **TONE/EXFOLIATE.** Use a cotton pad to apply a lactic acid exfoliating toner, using short upward strokes. Rinse.

3 **MOISTURIZE.** Layer on a thick moisturizer to finish up this routine. Look for ingredients like shea, hyaluronic acid, glycerin, aloe vera, and caprylic triglyceride that help lock in moisture by reducing water loss.

4 **APPLY SUNSCREEN** as you walk out the door

Broke B*tch

You don't have to spend a lot of money to have good skin. Using a combination of DIY, multifunction products, and a little creativity, you can have the glowy skin of a Nubian queen. A spa-grade turmeric mask can be whipped up in your kitchen, along with a luxurious body scrub.

Spending more doesn't always get you more. A lot of top-shelf products have the same formulations as your drugstore brands. If you come across an expensive product you like, take down the major ingredients and head to an outlet you can better afford. Odds are you can find something similar that will work for your wallet. There are some parts of your routine that are worth purchasing, like an all-season water-based cleanser and a protective sunscreen. The rest can be made in your kitchen. If you're looking for a full broke-b*tch routine, you've got it right here.

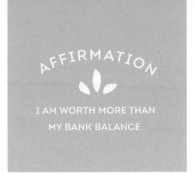

I AM WORTH MORE THAN
MY BANK BALANCE.

CLEANSE. Apply a gentle cleanser to your face, and work it into each area by moving three fingers in a circular motion.

TONE/EXFOLIATE. A combination toner and chemical exfoliating solution will give you bang for your buck. Gently pat the solution into your skin, covering your face, neck, and décolletage. Rinse as directed.

APPLY MASK. Choose your favorite DIY mask, starting on page 179.

MOISTURIZE. Coconut oil and olive oil can be repurposed as a moisturizer.

APPLY SUNSCREEN before you leave the house. This is not a product to cut, but a budget essential.

After a Breakup

You may have just lost a big part of your life, but you're still your best friend. Show up for yourself during this period of raw vulnerability by taking care of your skin. Breakups take many forms, but no matter what, they take a toll emotionally and sometimes even physically. The stress can show up as acne, or the crying can leave you feeling drained and dehydrated. Either way, any little bit you can do for yourself will go a long way. Reach out to your support network and invite them to mask and movie with you at home so you're feeling supported and rejuvenated at the same time.

AFFIRMATION

I AM GOING TO WORK THROUGH THE DISCOMFORT. I WILL IMMERSE MYSELF IN THE HEALING PROCESS. I HAVE THE POWER TO LIBERATE.

1 WRAP yourself in a warm blanket and call your best friend/mom.

2 MASSAGE. After shedding a few tears, you may experience some baggage, both emotional and physical, under your eyes. Use one of the de-puffing eye massages beginning on page 173.

3 APPLY MASK. You may not want to leave the house to buy a new sheet mask, so head to the kitchen. There are a few DIY mask recipes starting on page 179 that will give you a little project to distract yourself. Or pick your favorite mask and sluther it on.

4 SOAK. Emotions can be exhausting, and at this point, when you're neck-deep in your feels, you may not have the energy to do more than just lie down. So head to the bath and soak your body in a nutrient-rich and relaxing bath. You can find a few ideas beginning on page 170.

5 APPLY MASK ROUND 2. A hydrating squalane sleep mask will help your skin replenish its water loss from the tears you shed. There's no shame in crying, and honestly, it's too therapeutic not to. When you sleep tonight, coping may be a little easier if you know you're also taking part in self-care.

After a Day of Mansplaining

We all have those days. Someone, typically a man who has no idea what he's talking about, tries to explain to you how things work. You're the expert and yet, here you are, entertaining complete misinformation. The. Worst. On days like this, remind yourself that you are a queen, that your voice matters, and that you have enough self-respect to stand up for yourself. But all of that takes energy, and at the end of the day, you need to create space for yourself to restore and heal after such a taxing encounter. So light a candle, throw on a plush robe, and get into a little self-care.

AFFIRMATION

I AM A SMART, INSIGHTFUL POWERHOUSE. MY THOUGHTS ARE VALID, AND MY IDEAS DESERVE TO BE HEARD.

CLEANSE. Apply a gentle cleanser to your face, and work it into each area by moving three fingers in a circular motion.

APPLY MASK. Apply the soothing and hydrating yogurt shea mask found on page 185. If you're worried the stress from the day could lead to a breakout, go for a blemish care mask on page 180 instead.

SOAK. Take some extra time for yourself tonight and run a calming bath. It's a wonder what 15 minutes can do to relax your tense muscles and melt away the worries of the day.

SIP. Calming down before bed with a relaxing non-caffeinated tea will quench your soul and your thirst. After a warm bath, you'll want to hydrate with a glass of water because of all the water lost from sweating.

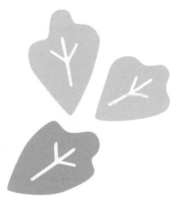

FOR THE GOOD TIMES

Lazy Sunday

Sunday is the one day of the week I keep exclusively for myself. If I can help it, I don't schedule any plans, work, or meetings for this day that don't contribute to my mental health or my love of unwinding. It's a practice that began when I was little. Growing up, my parents made it clear that it was the day of rest, a day to have lunch with the family, and for staying in the house outside of church service. Setting aside time for your self-care practice is a luxury, and if you can make it a whole day, even better. Take your time today and love on yourself—treat yourself right. You could even make yourself an extravagant meal or bake yourself something special. Beauty is inside and out, so on Sundays, let's tend to every part of ourselves.

AFFIRMATION

I AM MAKING SPACE FOR REFLECTION TODAY, TAKING WHAT I NEED TO DESIGN A THOUGHTFUL AND FULFILLING WEEK AHEAD.

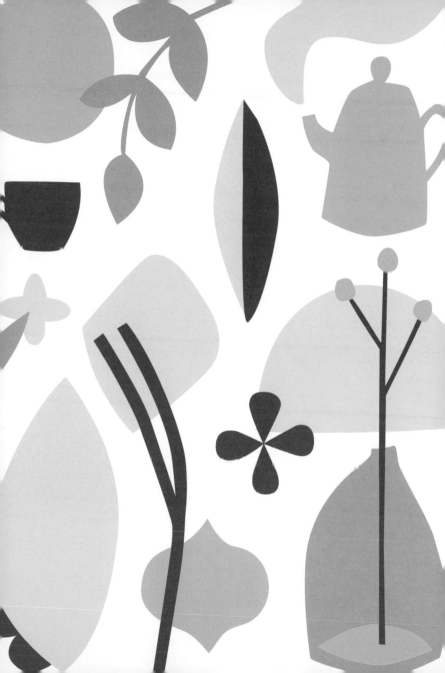

1 **HUMIDIFY.** Stand about 6 in (15 cm) away from a humidifier with a towel draped over your head and the steam vent to help channel the steam toward you for 5 minutes. If you don't have a humidifier, you can run a very hot shower and hang out in the steam or lay a steamy wash cloth (not too hot!) over your face. Applying steam to your face will begin the hydration process with nature's first beauty ingredient, H2O, and encourage sweat and toxins to move to the surface of your skin.

2 **CLEANSE.** Apply a gentle cleanser to your face, and work it into each area by moving three fingers in a circular motion, working your way from the inside out.

3 **SCRUB.** A simple sugar-based face scrub will quickly free you from dead skin and debris that may be nestled in the top layer of your skin. Be sure to apply this to your neck and décolletage, as well. These are areas that get less attention during the hustle and bustle of the weekday skin routine.

APPLY MASK. Use a charcoal-based mask to rebalance oil production and target any blemishes that may be on your face. It's also a great ingredient for skin that feels congested.

APPLY SECOND MASK. Make a custom mask for yourself this afternoon. Flip to page 179 for a few recipes. I suggest a soothing mask to indulge in while soaking in a bath.

SOAK. Take some extra time for yourself tonight and run a calming bath. It's a wonder what 15 minutes can do to relax your tense muscles and melt away the worries of the day.

MASSAGE. Take a few minutes to give yourself a thorough face massage. A few suggestions can be found starting on page 173.

Glass Slipper Sparkle

Your friends set you up on a big mystery date, and you're hoping he's heir to a big throne. So you want to sparkle like a jewel in the queen's crown. If things go well tonight, you may be showing a little more than just forearm to your new royal subject. Let's give you softened skin and a glow all over with a full-body scrub. You'll be so enthralled with how you feel after this, you might be more than content with just taking yourself home at the end of the night. Here's a quick refresh to get you prepped for a date.

AFFIRMATION

I AM A GEM WITH ENDLESS SPARKLE. NO ONE CAN EXTINGUISH MY LIGHT.

1 **CLEANSE.** Apply a gentle cleanser to your face, and work it into each area by moving three fingers in a circular motion.

2 **APPLY BODY SCRUB.** Step into the shower to keep this mess contained. Use a brown sugar scrub with a natural oil base to gently resurface your skin (like the one under Next Level on page 182). Start from the bottom with your feet, and gently work your way up. Spend about a minute on each section of your body to really dislodge the skin cells. Some areas may need more time. The whole process should take about 10 minutes. Then rinse and dry off. Be careful when getting out of the tub; it may be slippery with oil!

3 **APPLY MASK.** Apply a 24K gold mask, and leave it on as you get dressed and do your hair. It will leave you feeling like a precious metal. The gold will give you the firmness of youth and a lit-from-within glow. Leave on for 15 to 20 minutes.

4 **MOISTURIZE.** A shea-based moisturizing lotion or balm will effectively lock in moisture and condition the skin. It is particularly good at nourishing after a long, deep scrub.

Now you're the queen of the ball. Go get 'em!

Payday Coin Queen

Let's start by taking a second to admire those extra zeros in your account today. Money can't get you everything, but it can buy you some pretty luxurious skin-care products. So if you're ready to splurge on something extra for your skin, go for a mushy mask and a tool. Microcurrent tools—or as I refer to them, vibrators for your face—give you that all-too-good sensation to the touch and leave you with an enviable glow at the end. Spice things up with a new skin-care tool that keeps on giving. This routine is all about getting the most long-term value out of your routine and your paycheck.

AFFIRMATION

MY WEALTH IS WITHIN ME.
EVERY BREATH I TAKE SENDS MY
ENERGY OUT IN THE WORLD.

CLEANSE. Apply a gentle cleanser to your face, and work it into each area by moving three fingers in a circular motion.

 USE MICROCURRENT. Use your new microcurrent wand to exercise the muscles in your face and neck.

 APPLY MASK. Apply a 24K gold mask. It will leave you feeling like a precious metal. The gold will give you the firmness of youth and a lit-from-within glow. Leave on for 15 to 20 minutes.

MEDITATE. While money will cover you in gold, it means nothing without gratitude. Take a few minutes while you mask to meditate on some of the blessings in your life. I bet you can think of a few that won't fit in your wallet.

MOISTURIZE. A shea-based moisturizing lotion or balm will effectively lock in moisture and condition the skin. It is particularly good at nourishing and restoring the skin's natural barrier.

Picture Day

One of the most anxiety-inducing days of the year has got to be picture day. ID photos, yearbooks, company websites—these photos are the world's first impression of who you are, and you want them to be good. So that means no ultra-shiny forehead from the flash reflected off your face, less unwanted redness, and as few pimples as possible. A good rule of thumb is to stay away from astringent products or exfoliating the night before. This "night before" routine is all about soothing and calming the face to reduce the likelihood of capturing some less-than-desirable traits.

CLEANSE. Apply a gentle cleanser to your face, and work it into each area by moving three fingers in a circular motion.

APPLY MASK. Use a soothing DIY mask, like the ones on pages 184–185.

APPLY SERUM. Apply an evening primrose or jojoba oil serum. Both are soothing ingredients that have hydrating and anti-inflammatory properties, which are helpful for reducing the appearance of puffiness.

MOISTURIZE. A shea-based moisturizing lotion or balm will effectively lock in moisture and condition the skin. It is particularly good at nourishing and restoring the skin's natural barrier.

APPLY MASK. Use a hydrating sleep mask with aloe and glycerol overnight to make sure your face is fully moisturized when you wake up.

MASSAGE. In the morning, follow the Puff the Magic Dragon massage on page 176 to reduce any puffiness that may come from a great night's rest.

After a 3-Day Festival

Festivals filled with friends, live entertainment, and lots of booze are an essential summer event for many of us. But after a few days of nonstop action, your body needs some serious recovery time. Even your skin has a little bit of a hangover after an aggressive amount of alcohol consumption in such a small window of time. Drinking alcohol also reduces the protective shield around your skin's antioxidant network, which leaves you more exposed to the sun. If this is an outdoor daytime festival, you'll want to take extra precautions before and after.

Before:

1

WEAR SUNSCREEN. The best thing you can do for your skin is to just wear sunscreen, even if you do nothing else.

After:

CLEANSE. Use a water-based cleanser to remove the extra layer of sweat that has accumulated on your skin. Take your time and really work circles around your face. Create as much lather as you can before rinsing off. Lightly pat with a towel.

APPLY MASK AND SIP TEA. A deep-conditioning, hydrating mask will restore some of the water lost from having the time of your life and that alcohol consumption. While your mask sets, drink a little "beauty tea" to get your voice back from all the screaming. I recommend a ginger tea with a hint of lemon and honey.

APPLY SERUM. Apply 3 to 4 drops of hemp or rosehip oil. The nourishing omega-3 fatty acids will repair the extra sun damage you likely racked up over the last few days.

MOISTURIZE. Choose a moisturizer with squalane. Squalane is helpful for regulating oil production while also hydrating the skin. Take a quarter-size portion into your palm and rub your hands together. Gently work the moisturizer into your face, making sure to cover every surface.

MASSAGE YOUR EYES. Exercise the muscles around your eyes with the invigorating massage on page 175. This will bring more circulation to the area, as well.

AFFIRMATION

TODAY I AM BALANCING MY
ENERGY, RIDING THE HIGHS,
AND EMBRACING THE CALM.

Before Brunch with the Girls

There's nothing like getting together with the girls over some Eggs Benedict and a tofu scramble. Your best friends are always looking out for you, which means they'll notice if your skin is looking dull because they're worried about you. Bellinis are so much more delicious when the conversation is about why your skin is glowing on a Sunday morning. To get that glow, let's focus on exfoliating to reduce the appearance of dullness and to add some dewy magic.

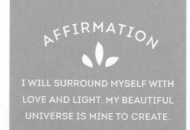

AFFIRMATION

I WILL SURROUND MYSELF WITH LOVE AND LIGHT. MY BEAUTIFUL UNIVERSE IS MINE TO CREATE.

1 CLEANSE with an oil cleanser.

2 EXFOLIATE. A sugar-based exfoliating scrub will resurface your skin and give it a fresh glow. Removing that top layer of dead or dying skin cells is the fastest way to relieve dullness.

3 APPLY SERUM. Apply 3 to 4 drops of a carrot seed serum to your face. Carrot seed oil can give you a revitalized glow while also packing in serious antioxidant properties, which are important for a long-term glow.

 MOISTURIZE. Apply a quarter-size amount of a squalane gel moisturizer to your face. A lightweight gel moisturizer will give you that dewy appearance because its texture allows it to live as a thin layer on your face while it delivers the active ingredients to your skin.

5 MIST. Spritz a light hydrating mist 2 to 3 times and lightly pat the solution onto your face. Now, brunch!

BATHING: A MASK FOR THE REST OF YOUR SKIN

Bathleisure is the ultimate lifestyle. In fact, on my last apartment leasing adventure, it was on the top of my priority list, because there is nothing like coming home from a long day, running a bath, and soaking as your face mask sets. Let the bathtub be your happy place, a sanctuary for self-care and self-love. There's something so purifying and even spiritual about stepping into the water with your worries and then leaving feeling cleansed of them. I've talked a lot about taking care of the skin on your face and neck because it is a big part of your identity and what people see. But there are so many private parts of us, the inner parts that also need tending to, and a bath is the perfect place to make that happen.

The Relax-Her
(Milk, Honey, Ginger)

Milk baths have been the soaking base of choice for several ancient royals, like Napoleon's sister Pauline; Roman empresses; and even Queen Elizabeth I. These women bathed in milk because they believed it had ethereal powers of beautification and healing. The Old French, Greek, and Latin variations of baptism—*baptisier*, *baptizein*, and *baptizare*—all agree that it is an experience of whole body immersion and cleansing. Egyptian Pharaoh Cleopatra believed so deeply in the disease-healing power of donkey's milk that herds of donkeys were raised just so she could bathe regularly. The power of soaking has been acknowledged as both a physical and mental rehabilitation; and I encourage you to integrate it into your self-care routine.

1   Fill your tub with medium warm water.

2   Mix in 1 cup [125 g] of milk powder or 2 cups [480 ml] of your favorite milk

3   Add 2 Tbsp of honey.

4   Add 3 dashes of ground ginger.

5   Mix and soak for 20 to 30 minutes or until you get pruney.

Detox (Bentonite Clay, Green Tea, Epsom Salts)

If a milk bath doesn't fit in to your self-care practice, you can also stick with a water-based bath that takes advantage of some natural antioxidants. Sitting in the warm water of a bath will cause your body to start sweating, and that is the first form of detoxification. Bentonite clay and green tea aid in this process as natural antioxidants and detoxifiers. Adding Epsom salts to any bath will help relax tense muscles after a workout or just a very long day. Take a load off and let the healing waters do their thing.

1   Dissolve ½ cup [70 g] of bentonite clay powder into 3 cups of water.

2   Pour bentonite mixture into a warm water bath.

3   Steep 2 bags of green tea in the bath.

4   (Optional) Add a handful of Epsom salts.

5   Soak for half an hour and live your best life.

AFTER BATHING: You'll want to drink a lot of water if you used hot water for your bath because it can be quite dehydrating. Think about it. You just sweated out a lot of stress in that hot bath. You'll need a drink to replace all that water loss. Finish up with an oil rub, balm, or lotion that contains coconut oil, which is highly compatible with the skin and very moisturizing.

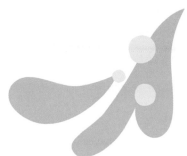

FACIAL MASSAGES

If you ever feel like your face is bloated or congested, you're not alone. Often this is because of poor drainage from your lymph nodes. Your body is very good at detoxing, and all that material ends up in your lymph nodes. To give you a brief human anatomy lesson, the *lymph nodes* are the tiny ducts that collect the white blood cells and debris resulting from an infection. You'll typically feel your lymph nodes swell and feel tender to the touch when fighting off the flu or the common cold. That's not the only time they're working. Your body is constantly working to get rid of any toxins or unrecognized agents that may be wreaking havoc. The lymph nodes collect and filter lymph fluid, which contains white blood cells, proteins, bacteria, and fats. Lymph nodes are scattered throughout your body, but several of them are in your face. You can help this drainage process along by massaging and applying pressure on what I call the sweet spots. The feeling is similar to massaging aching muscles after a tough workout. That "hurts so good" delicious sensation is what we'll be going for with these massages. They also double as tension-relievers, as many of us hold stress in the muscles of our face. Take a moment and relax.

Micromanage Draining

This mini massage will help drain some of the lymphatic fluids that build up under your eyes and at the sides of your face. It's short and sweet, but you'll feel brand-new. Take a break from your day and handle some personal business.

WHAT YOU NEED: FRESH AIR; BEST IF YOUR EYES ARE CLOSED.

1   Place your middle finger at the intersection of your eyebrows and the bridge of your nose. Move up to your hairline, applying medium pressure. Repeat 3 times.

2   Press your thumbs in between your eyebrows and outward toward your temples, tracing your eyebrows with your fingers. Repeat 3 times.

3   Press your pointer and middle fingers just below your tear ducts and move outward. Repeat 5 to 7 times.

4   Press your pointer and middle fingers to your temples and move down over your neck. Repeat 5 times.

Caught the Red-Eye

This under-eye massage is a quick refresher that you can whip out in the course of a busy day or after a late night. Puffiness can be a giveaway that you don't have it all together, so here we're focusing on reducing that inflammation and some slight lymphatic drainage. We're going to start with our focus just under the eye, where you might find a dark circle on tough days.

WHAT YOU NEED: MOISTURIZER OR EYE CREAM; COMPASSION FOR YOURSELF.

1   Take your moisturizer or eye cream and dab a little bit onto each middle finger.

2   Using gentle pressure, starting near your tear ducts and moving outward, dab your fingertips around the contour of the bottom lids, creating a string of pearls with the moisturizer. Stop just before you reach your temples. Repeat 3 times.

3   Go back over that line with light pressure, but this time in long sweeping motions, to connect the dots. Repeat 3 times.

4   Breathe in, breathe out. You can do this.

Puff the Magic Dragon

This massage will reduce puffiness in your face. I recommend doing this in the morning before you start your day or if you find yourself getting puffy during the day. I always feel relief in my face after this massage.

WHAT YOU NEED: A LIGHT OIL OR SERUM; A LITTLE SELF-LOVE.

1 Rub a few drops of serum into your hands and wrists. Take your triple threat fingers (middle, ring, and pinky) on each hand and place them on each side of your forehead, right near the hairline. Apply medium to light pressure as you move them downward toward your ears. Repeat 5 times.

2 Use those same triple threat fingers and place them at the middle of your forehead. Move them outward toward your temples. Repeat 5 times.

3 Place your thumbs at the inner pocket of your brows; each should be flanking the bridge of your nose. Hold your thumbs in place and apply light pressure for 5 counts; then sweep your thumbs across your eyelids. This is my favorite step. Repeat 3 times or as needed.

4 Place your triple threat fingers at the base of your nose and on either side of your lips. Apply medium pressure as you move them in the shape of a C up toward your temples. Repeat 5 times.

5 Place your wrists between your chin and your bottom lip. Apply medium pressure upward in the shape of a C, starting just below your cheekbones, and moving toward your temples. Lean your head forward for a more intense effect Repeat 3 to 5 times.

6 Place your index and middle fingers at the top of your forehead. Apply medium pressure as you move them around the sides of your face and down through your neck. Repeat 3 to 5 times.

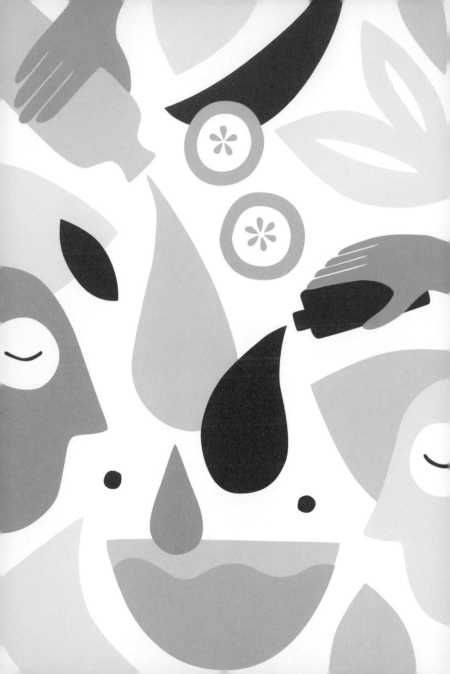

DIY MASK RECIPES

Blemish Care: Coffee Culture Mask

Coffee culture is undeniable and inescapable around the world. Rubbing coffee onto your skin can give you a lit-from-within glow while exfoliating and reinvigorating your skin (and finding a use for those coffee grounds). On top of that, this is a great mask for dealing with blemishes that are looking large and angry from inflammation.

An exfoliating mask like this coffee-based mixture will re-surface the skin and remove dead cells. This is important for managing hyperpigmentation that might result from acne and scars left behind by former breakouts. Leave on for 10 to 15 minutes, and be sure to scrub the full surface of your face before rinsing off. Glow.

INGREDIENTS

½ CUP [54 G] PRE-USED, DAMP COFFEE GROUNDS
¼ CUP [60 G] YOGURT
2 TSP GROUND TURMERIC

Blemish Care: Manuka Honey Mask

Manuka honey is a natural antimicrobial agent with incredible healing powers for your skin. It hails from Australia and New Zealand, where the bees seem to exude their own special glow. The manuka bush produces flowers that when used to make honey have four times the mineral power compared to regular honey. That makes this superfood rich in iron, manganese, zinc, and more. For centuries it has been applied to fresh wounds to prevent infection and reduce the inflammatory response from a cut or burn. It lowers the pH of the wound, which is important for restoring the skin's natural pH of about 5.5. Honey is also a humectant, which means that it prevents the loss of water from the surface of your skin.

Another potent ingredient in this mask is bentonite clay. This ingredient is important for drying out blemishes and encouraging the release of toxins that may be on the face. When combined with honey, you get a multifaceted approach to reducing inflammation, drying out pimples, and hydrating your skin.

You can use this mask as a spot treatment or as a full-on mask. Leave on for 10 to 15 minutes.

INGREDIENTS

½ CUP [70 G] BENTONITE CLAY POWDER
1 TO 2 TBSP OLIVE OIL (ADJUST FOR CONSISTENCY)
1 TBSP MANUKA HONEY
2 TSP GROUND TURMERIC

Rosacea: Redness-Reducing Mask

Kanuka honey (not to be confused with manuka honey) hails from New Zealand, and it has been scientifically and clinically proven to treat rosacea when applied as a face mask. Use this recipe twice a week to reap the full benefits of this antimicrobial and anti-inflammatory agent. Managing the inflammatory response of rosacea will also reduce the outward redness. During a rosacea flare-up, inflammation leads to *vasodilation*, the enlarging of blood vessels that leads to redness as blood rushes to the face. A simultaneous breakdown of the collagen around these blood vessels is like a double whammy that weakens blood vessels and brings more blood to the face.

Enter the super ingredient kanuka honey with naturally potent anti-inflammatory properties, making it the perfect alternative approach to rosacea. If you're hoping for a solution to your rosacea that will not contribute to the rise of antibiotic resistance, then this grocery store product will do the trick. Leave on for 15 to 20 minutes.

INGREDIENTS

2 TBSP KANUKA HONEY
1 TSP GLYCERIN
PINCH OF GROUND CINNAMON
1 TBSP FRESHLY SQUEEZED LEMON JUICE

NEXT LEVEL: You can turn this mask into a scrub by adding ½ cup [100 g] of brown sugar and a ½ tablespoon of olive oil. Mix until you get a medium to thick consistency. Adjust proportions to suit your needs.

Soothing Mask:
Yogurt + Clay

Greek yogurt is a dairy queen's dream masking ingredient.
Not only does it have the all-around good-for-you properties
of a probiotic, but the instant cooling effect it has on the skin
is hard to beat. Leave on for 10 to 15 minutes.

INGREDIENTS

½ CUP [120 G] YOGURT
½ CUP [70 G] BENTONITE CLAY POWDER
1 TSP ROSEHIP OIL (CAN BE YOUR SERUM)

Soothing Mask: Yogurt + Shea

Shea butter is near and dear to my heart. It originates from western and central Africa, where the mangifolia tree reigns as the tree of life. That name is well deserved given the immense number of significant benefits that shea butter brings. A cocktail of vitamins E, A, K, and F make it a super ingredient that heals wounds, softens the skin's texture, hydrates, and packs a ton of antioxidants. My mother recently brought me back a tub of raw shea butter fresh from Africa (she picked it up in Cameroon) and I've been able to use it in so many ways, one of which is a mask that I'll share here. If you aren't lucky enough to be able to get raw shea butter straight from the source, you can still find plenty of ways to buy it online. Leave on for 10 to 15 minutes.

INGREDIENTS

½ CUP [123 G] YOGURT
2 TSP SHEA BUTTER
2 DROPS OF YOUR FAVORITE MOISTURIZING SERUM

Acknowledgments

My story is an unconventional one. My grandparents were illiterate farmers in central Africa, where my parents were both born. I was born in Antwerp, Belgium, and my first language was Flemish. When we moved to the United States, I had to figure out how to communicate with my new peers and find my voice again. As the oldest of four and the child of immigrants, I had to figure out how to make my dreams come true. When my dad became ill and ultimately passed away, it felt like I had lost my way once again, like I was that little girl who spoke Dutch when all the kids spoke English.

Well, these people stepped in and showed me the way. They reminded me of my strength, my dreams, and my power: Thank you to my mother who, despite her better judgment, did not disown me when I decided to turn down medical school and write a skin care book instead. She has been a relentless supporter of my dreams, rough-around-the-edges spirit, and many compulsive decisions. From her I learned what true strength is, and for all the days of my life, I will be trying to grow into someone half as strong as her.

Greg, my greatest love. Your endless, irrational, and unconditional support of all my endeavors has given me the strength to live life fearlessly. Thank you for kicking me out of bed early in the morning to meet my book deadlines and sacrificing countless nights of rest and peace while enduring my crazy and inexplicable writing habits. You are my person.

Tomi, my dearest friend, sister, and ride or die. We've laughed, cried, danced, and supported each other through incredible highs and devastating lows. Thank you for telling me what I already knew, but refused to believe—that my path was still forming and greatness was on it. But also, thank you for being a freaking badass at everything you do, forcing me to level up. As you well know, African languages matter. . .

Lanya Olmsted, my partner in crime and lifelong work wife. You make every day an unforgettable adventure. Thank you for taking a leap with me, a gift that I will forever be grateful for. From your creativity to your intuition to your incredible talent, you have taught me more about being a partner than I could have ever imagined. You once told me, "Your skin is a reflection of who you surround yourself with and what you put inside your body. Take care, lovely skin, take care." And I live that truth every day I come to work.

Yasmin Rawlins, remember when we first met, in the library, delirious yet full of hope? You help me believe that I can live and thrive as my fullest, most authentic self. Thank you for always being there.

Jasmine Wyatt, thank you for serving in our nation's capital at a time when our country needs, but could not possibly deserve, unwaveringly dedicated citizen-leaders like you. And thank you for accepting that this baby dragon could be a good friend. You're my family and I love you.

Heather Buffo, my cheerleader and favorite blonde. Thank you for your constant thoughtfulness, for your spirited support, and for leaving me the world's best phone messages. Don't get upset, but you'll probably read this just before or after one of your frequent showers.

Jennifer Sunmonu, or Jenny (yes, I just called you that), thank you for rooting for me, giggling with me, and saying yes to so many of my crazy ideas. I think your witchy powers are starting to rub off on me.

To my editor, Deanne, who I first thought was an internet scammer. Thank you for sending me that Instagram message and changing my life. Little did you know, that message led me to upend my life and pursue a dream that I thought would never leave the depths of my nighttime slumber. For the gentle respect with which you listened to my needs, the care with which you read my fervent words, and the ruthlessness with which you edited this book into something people would actually love, you were the best partner in bringing this to life.

To my dad, who told me years ago that the most important skill I could develop was communication. He said that being smart is one thing, but it is nothing if you can't share your knowledge with others. He also frequently reminded me that I didn't need any adornments and that my natural state was my most beautiful. Thank you for showing me that I had a glow.

Index

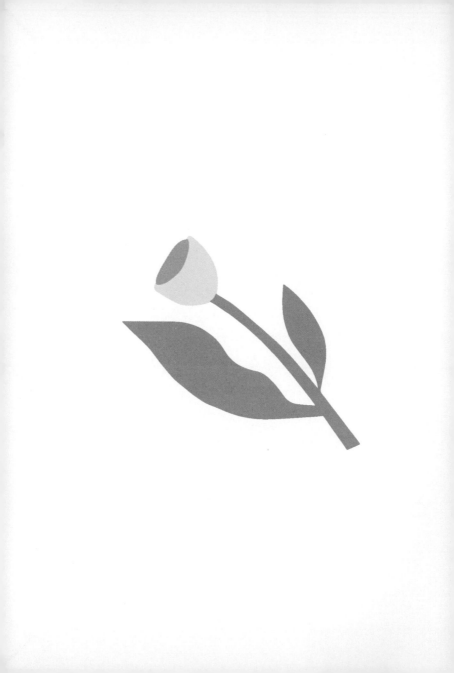